It's Okay to Laugh

to Laugh

(Crying Is Cool Too)

It's Okay to Laugh

to Laugh

(Crying Is Cool Too)

A memoir about
loving madly and
letting go

Nora McInerny Purmort

piatkus

PIATKUS

First published in the US in 2016 by HarperCollins
First published in Great Britain in 2016 by Piatkus

Copyright © 2016 Nora McInerny Purmort

Designed by Shannon Nicole Plunkett

1 3 5 7 9 10 8 6 4 2

A CIP catalogue record for this book
is available from the British Library.

ISBN 978-0-349-41012-8

Printed and bound in Great Britain by
Clays Ltd, St Ives plc

Papers used by Piatkus are from well-managed forests
and other responsible sources.

 MIX
Paper from
responsible sources
FSC® C104740

Piatkus
An imprint of
Little, Brown Book Group
Carmelite House
50 Victoria Embankment
London EC4Y 0DZ

An Hachette UK Company

www.hachette.co.uk

This is a collection of stories about my life, told the way I remember them, after losing a couple hundred brain cells. I changed some names, but not all of them. If you remember these stories differently, good for you!

For Aaron.

Us.

For Steve.

Semper Fi.

Contents

Introduction

You are holding a book by another youngish white woman who had a pretty charmed life until her father and husband died of cancer a few weeks after she miscarried her second baby. That's just the truth: 2014 sucked pretty hard, but for most of my life, things were easy. I have three siblings and we are all (currently) on speaking terms. I was voted Most Likely to Have a Talk Show in high school. My parents mostly loved and respected each other, even if my dad referred to my beautiful, thin mother as Large Marge. My grandparents died when they were old, so I was sad but okay with it. I got to go to private school from kindergarten to college and I don't even have student loans to pay off. Seriously, how much do you hate me right now?

But easy as things were, I was always certain that I was somehow wasting time, that everything was slipping through my fingers and I was never going to do anything with my one wild and precious life. I kept waiting for someone else to tell me how to do it. It seemed like everyone else always knew what they were doing . . . but how? How did they know who to marry and how to get a car loan, or what number to put for their tax deductions so their parents wouldn't end up paying their income taxes during their first year of "adulthood"? Where was the life syllabus, and how did I miss it?

Now I am a thirty-two-year-old widowed mom and I don't have time to worry about whether or not I'm doing it right, because I *know* that my one wild and precious life is indeed slipping through my hands. If I want to do something Big and Important, I have to do it before five o'clock because day care is strict about pickup time. I'm not so worried anymore, because now I know *nobody* knows what they are doing in life, and *nobody* knows what to do when bad things happen, to themselves or to other people. We make it up as we go, and sometimes we are big and generous and sometimes we are small and petty. We say the wrong things, we obsess over all the ways we got it wrong and all the ways that other people did, too. The only thing I know for sure is that it is okay not to know everything, to try and to fail and to sometimes suck at life, as long as you try to get better.

I'm not writing this book to bum you out, although parts of it are for sure a bummer. I'm thinking specifically about the parts where my dad dies, or my husband dies, or I miscarry a baby. I don't need your pity—I have plenty of my own, and I spend it creating sad stories about old men I see alone at the bus stop. I am writing it because bad stuff is like good stuff: it just happens.

People really expect that huge life events will make you older and wiser, and in some ways, they do. I now have a will! I don't give all the fucks about what people say about me on the Internet! And in some ways, I came out of these events like any other person: a little irritated at how many people complain about cold and flu season like they were just diagnosed with Stage IV brain cancer, and a little preoccupied with how flat my butt looks since I had a child.

I'm writing a book about it—the good stuff and the terrible stuff—because I know I'm not special. This stuff happens to everyone. I'm not an expert on grief or parenting or even writing (maybe I Googled "How to Write a Book," maybe not; who's to say?). I am just another dummy with a blog and a collection of Most Improved awards from her days as a mediocre high school athlete, trying every day to get better at life. Not every life lesson comes from death and tragedy: sometimes it comes from flipping off your high school principal because he was illegally driving in the carpool lane.

This is for people who have been through some shit—or have watched someone go through it. This is for people who aren't sure if they're saying or doing the right thing (you're not, but nobody is). This is for people who had their life turned upside down and just learned to live that way. For people who have laughed at a funeral or cried in a grocery store. This is for everyone who wondered what exactly they're supposed to be doing with their one wild and precious life. I don't actually have the answer, but if you find out, will you text me?

Chapter 1

Lay Off Me, Mary

Tell me, what is it you plan to do with
your one wild and precious life?
—MARY OLIVER

Umm, I don't know, Mary. I'm not great at planning, can't I
just go with the flow? Honestly, this little quote stresses me
out sometimes. It's like YOLO for women with Pinterest.

My life is wild and precious. I only have one. What am I going
to do with it? Well, for starters, I'm going to do so many things I
never wanted to do. I'm going to play sports I don't even like just
because I'm tall. Even as a grown-up, years after my last game, I
will say "yep" when old men ask if I play basketball just because I
don't want to disappoint them. I'm going to be mean just to fit in.
I'm going to tip waitresses 20 percent even when they are mean to
me. I'm going to live with a thin little skin, where I let every insult

wound me and every compliment slide right off my back. I think I am doing this wrong.

I will be stressed to the max, Mary. Even when I'm a kid. I'm going to be certain that every paper I write will be the one that determines my future.

In the summertime, I will go to Lake Superior with my brother and my cousins. I will float in the icy water and imagine I am a tiny pebble. I will swim until my lips are blue.

I will play the saxophone for a whole year and nobody in my family will remember. This will annoy me because who lies about playing the saxophone?

I will forgive my uncle when he calls me, a seven-year-old, impersonates Goofy, and tells me I've won a trip to Disneyland.

I will go to Disneyland—as an adult. My husband and I will watch the haggard couples screaming at each other over their strollers. We will hold the sweaty little hands of our niece and nephew and purchase overpriced souvenir ears and limp salads. That night, in the dark of our hotel room, we will decide to have a baby together. Cancer be damned, whatever it takes.

I will say the f-word even after I'm sent to my room for shouting it when my little brother breaks my tailbone in a wrestling match for the remote control when we are both in high school. One day, while I am changing his diaper, my two-year-old son, Ralph, will smile, look me right in the eye, and say, "Oh, fuck!" And I will laugh.

I'm going to make sure I spend most of my college experience stumbling drunk through the streets of Cincinnati. Or, better yet, being pushed around in a stolen grocery cart. I will know I am wasting this opportunity, so I will try to keep that feeling quiet. I will try to starve it away, or push it down with hours in the gym. I will let my jeans slide on and off without unbuttoning them. I will count my ribs with my fingers at night.

I will spend years mimicking the fashion stylings of Britney Spears: pierced belly button with a hot pink jewel, tanning-bed tan, and chunky highlights. When she and Justin Timberlake break up, I will cry in my dorm room and wonder if love is even real.

I will listen to a friend tell me about having sex in the basement of a party with a senior. When I repeat the story to my boyfriend, who is halfway across the country at a small liberal arts college where he takes women's studies and plays football, he will say, "That's not sex, that's rape," and I will know he is right but not what to do about it.

A very important thing to do with your wild and precious life is to get a job, so I will do that. I will sit in a cubicle, I suppose. And then another cubicle. I'd always imagined a really stately office with lots of books, but this beige little pen will do just fine. It comes with a wastebasket! And a little sorter thing for all my folders, which I will never use because that's what a computer does now. I will make a lot of PowerPoint documents about very important "strategies" for things like how a "consumer" can "connect" with a fossil fuels brand on Twitter, because you know what? That's all people want to do these days. They're just opening up Twitter hoping to start a dialogue with the guys who put the gas in their SUVs. And I can say I helped make that happen, Mary. Isn't *that* something?

I will sometimes hate-read blogs written by people I despise, just to make my blood boil. You probably don't hate-read anything because you have a sparkling mind that has not been pecked to death by the incessant information assault that is the Internet. But seriously, Mary, how many lifestyle blogs does the world need? How many photos of coffee? How many hashtags do we need on one photo and can't we just have a brunch without labeling all the beverages with small chalk signs, Mary?? Can't we?

Sometimes I will read Twitter right when I wake up, when only one of my eyes opens fully. I will follow hashtags that make me want to punch someone. I'm talking about you, #notallmen, #meninism, and #alllivesmatter.

I will fall in love, quickly the first time, and slower every time after that. "I hope we are in love FOREVER," I will write in my bubbly, high-school-girl handwriting.

I will say "I love you" when I don't exactly mean it, but "I love you" sounds better than "You are my best option at the time, though I know you have reached your full potential and I am destined for greater things, buddy." That's okay, right?

I will choose the wrong man sometimes. All right, most of the time. Okay, every time except once or twice.

I will sometimes miss these men who were not right for me. I will think of them when I hear certain songs by long-lost indie bands, or smell marijuana in the summertime. I will always say it wasn't love, but it was. Love is not always perfect, is it, Mary? Isn't it sometimes awkward and bumbling?

I will move to New York for love. I won't have a job, or any money, but I will feel very alive and very special and cosmopolitan even though "date night" sometimes means eating at Olive Garden in Times Square, because I am dating a man who is comfortable enough to admit that his favorite kind of Italian food is "Italian food."

I will learn the words to misogynistic rap songs, even though I am a feminist. I will always turn it down when my car rolls up beside an elderly person.

Sometimes I will be small and mean and ugly and jealous.

Sometimes I will be open and loving and generous.

I will do anything to avoid being lonely. I will wake up in beds where I do not belong, grab my things, and go.

I will pick my nose and hope nobody is looking.

I will judge other people, and find myself doing nearly all those things I judged them for. See: my giant, all-terrain stroller; handing my child an iPhone to keep him quiet when we are out to dinner and he is losing his mind; co-sleeping with him until he is thirty (fingers crossed).

I will choose the right man when it really matters. I will tell him once that it is my dream to be on the kiss cam, and at every sporting event, he will conspire to make sure we make out hardcore every time the Jumbotron camera passes by us. I will watch him die in my arms. I'm not saying that to be dramatic, I'm saying it because aside from pushing a live baby out of my hidey-hole it is the most meaningful thing I *have* done with this wild and precious life. I will tell our son that his papa is in his heart, and in mine. Like the word "fuck," Ralph will remember that. He will remind me on gray spring days when I am wiping his lunch from the floor, where he's been so kind as to sprinkle it. "My papa loves you," he'll say to me, with his crooked-teeth grin, "he's in my heart."

I'll be quick to forget everything good I've ever done. I will replay every time I have ever been an asshole, and hate myself for every wrong thing I've ever said and done.

Yes, it stressed me out to be asked about my plans for my one— ONE—wild and precious life, but I will still like this phrase every time someone has turned it into art on Pinterest or Instagram. I will try not to let it stress me out. I will try to be better. I will try to bring more love to the world.

Chapter 2

Now

"I don't want to have cancer," he whispers. We are curled up in his hospital bed, trying to go to sleep in the alternate universe we've found ourselves in. When we woke up this morning, we were just a regular young couple secretly cohabitating after a year of dating. But somewhere in the middle of the day, he'd had a seizure, ended up in the hospital, and found out he'd somehow grown a brain tumor without even noticing.

"You don't have cancer," I tell him, because he doesn't. He has a tumor. And until they open up his head to take it out, that tumor could be anything: a conjoined twin absorbed into his skull at birth, a silver dollar, a handful of cotton candy.

But it's not cancer. Because I won't let it be, and in my twenty-eight years on this earth I've become goddamn used to getting whatever the hell I want. My first boyfriend, an A when I deserved a B in American history junior year of high school, my first job, the dimple in my right cheek. That's just a sampling of the things I've gotten through sheer willpower.

Whatever the nurse gave Aaron a few minutes ago is starting to work, and I can feel his body gently relax next to me. I'd asked if I could have a sleeping aid, too, but Nurse Neil just laughed and dropped his signature line, "I know, right?" so I'm left wide awake in the glow of my boyfriend's heart monitor. I keep my hand on his head and my head on his heart and in the glow of our new night-light I command the universe to keep going my way.

And then I am standing by his grave, having traveled at light speed from the present to the worst-case scenario. The priest is swinging incense over Aaron's body, I am kneeling next to his mother in a church pew, I am throwing a handful of damp earth onto his casket, shiny as a Cadillac.

We are young and in love, and my boyfriend is going to die.

He will die, I know it, and I go there, though I have no business doing so. Our human imaginations are woefully unprepared for predicting actual pain, but I hack away at it anyway, trying to form a scar before I am even wounded.

November has always been the cruelest month. November is gray and stark, each day growing shorter and shorter until December can plunge us into total darkness. November took my uncle and my grandmother and many years after we've laid them each to rest, when the sting of this month has become more of a dull ache, November is trying to claim Aaron.

As a child, I was always worried that my parents would die if I slept away from our home, because I was a very normal and happy child with no anxiety issues at all.

Sleepovers were rare, because my father was strict and old-fashioned and believed that a child belonged in her bed and not on the floor of some half-finished Minneapolis basement watching PG-13 movies and getting made fun of for her headgear, but they did happen, and I'd always spend the night racked with insomnia, imagining the demise of my parents and my impending orphanhood.

One by one, my friends would drift off to sleep, and I would lay awake among them, imagining my older sister delivering the news when I walked into our home the next day with my sleeping bag under my arm, and calling out to our family, "Yoo hoo!" in imitation of our now dead mother. I pictured my siblings and myself lined up in the front row of the church, kneeling before our parents' coffins in coordinating all-black outfits. My brothers would offer me their handkerchiefs to dry my tears. My brothers would apparently have handkerchiefs.

There would be a custody battle, of course. We'd all be split among our godparents—that's what godparents do, right? Just take over when your parents die in a sleepover-related accident?—and that would be the end of our family. All because I needed to sleep at Catherine's house and chat on AIM with strangers.

My parents never did die (or, my dad did, but later, and of cancer, and that wasn't my fault, I wasn't at a sleepover) but I replayed these scenes all the time throughout my childhood, a way of trying on feelings and situations that didn't fit yet, that wouldn't for years to come.

But this is different. This is fucking wrong.

It is wrong to try on this fictitious sorrow for size when Aaron is sleeping beside me, and I drag myself from this imaginary hell into the real and present one in front of me, sneaking out of our hospital bed to wash my hot, tear-soaked face with cool water and look into my own tired eyes in the tiny, beige-tiled, fluorescent-lit en suite bathroom in his hospital room. There are two tiny soaps that you know will instantly turn your skin to sandpaper, plain toothbrushes with bristles so weak it's like brushing your teeth with baby hair, and a small bottle of lotion that smells like gasoline. If you had a really excellent imagination and a really bad sense of what a hotel experience should be like, you could almost pretend you were at a cheap motel, though even those don't have ball-chain cords next to the toilet to pull in case of emergency.

Aaron was where I'd left him, sleeping on his side in a hospital bed built for one, leaving space for me. *You cannot do that again,* I tell myself. *You cannot bury the man you love while he is still alive.*

So I didn't. I fought the urge to try to feel things before they happened and instead tried to feel what was actually happening. I think this is called "being present" or "living your life" but it was a really new concept for me, and it blew my mind in the same way discovering that Lumiere in *Beauty and the Beast* is voiced by Jerry Orbach from *Law & Order,* or that Drake was Jimmy on *Degrassi.* Aaron had brain surgery and got discharged from the hospital and we went to the supermarket Target, as is customary. He was diagnosed with brain cancer and we decided to get married, like, immediately, cancer be damned. We didn't spend time reading about brain tumors or bothering with statistics because fuck it, we had several HBO series to watch, and that didn't leave a lot of time for worrying. We got so good at being alive in the moment that I think a lot of people in our lives forgot Aaron was sick. And actually, I think we sometimes forgot Aaron was sick, and that an incurable cancer meant an impossible future. But who needed the future? Until we'd have to wake up at 6:00 A.M. for an MRI or go see his oncologist, we were just a regular young couple who had more chemo than food in their cupboards and were on a first-name basis with the radiation staff.

A day before our wedding, I had one small word tattooed in cursive inside my right wrist. It was my "something new" for our wedding day, and a reminder to myself that nothing good ever came of time traveling.

It's just one tiny word that helped me do the biggest things in life, like getting married and buying a house and having a baby or getting my ears pierced at age thirty-two. I look at it every day, to remind me what time it is: *now*.

Chapter 3
Stories

There's very little that makes me as sad as seeing a couple sitting silently at dinner, pushing their food around their plates or ignoring one another in favor of the cool glow of their phones.

I'm not talking about the quiet rhythms of a loving relationship, or the nights where you and your dining partner agree to tandem-eavesdrop on your table neighbors in order to fully understand just whose brother slept with the other's wife while he was in jail. I'm talking about two people who love each other out at dinner having separate dates with their iPhones, who find reading tweets from strangers more interesting than the person who knows them best.

I promised myself a long time ago that I would never be that person, that I would never resign myself to a relationship where there was a possibility that you could ever run out of things to talk about.

That is perhaps the defining characteristic that distinguishes my relationship with Aaron from my relationship with any other boy, man, or man-child: Aaron always had a story to tell, and always wanted to listen to my own.

We started our daily ritual on the first night I spent at his house: my head on his bony chest, drifting into the first stages of sleep while he told me about The Time a Kid Threw a Bees' Nest at Another Kid at the Bus Stop or The Time He Fell Through the Ceiling at the Movie Theater or The Time His Mother Tried to Teach Him to Drive a Stick Shift.

In turn, I knew I could tell him anything, always. And I did. I told him about The Time I Threw Up All My Food for a Year and The Time I Started Smoking So a Boy Would Like Me (He Didn't) and The Time I Threw Up in My Hands and Pooped My Pants: A College Horror Story. Why are all my stories about vomit?

We do this every night after that first one. Or we try to. I usually request one of his greatest hits and then fall asleep halfway through with my mouth open so he gets a long, sexy look at my retainer. But one night, he is more tired than usual and wants me to do the talking.

"Tell me something I don't know about you yet," he whispers. So I do.

I don't know why it comes to mind, but I tell him about the time when I was ten when two of my friends spent a day passing me mean notes, little bombs of bitchiness folded into perfect squares and dropped onto my lap or my desk between lessons.

Are you still on the swim team? Is it the chlorine that makes you so ugly?

Why are you so annoying? Do you know why everyone hates you?

In their defense, I *was* ugly, and the chlorine wasn't helping matters much. And I don't know why I was so annoying, I just was, okay?

I spent the day feeling sad and embarrassed and small and the next day, for reasons I'll never understand, I paid the favor forward and started passing mean notes to my best friend, just to see what it felt like to be on the other side.

It felt shitty, of course. But not as shitty as when she told her mother, who told my mother, who gave me the kind of look that affirms that you are indeed a piece of human garbage who should go spend some introspective time writing in her diary about the time she made her best friend feel like shit.

I hate this memory, but I pull it out anyway, hand over hand, until all the shame around it dislodges inside me and lays on the bed between us. I can see even in the dark that he's aghast.

"That's horrible," he says, because all his stories are funny, and because it is, and together we both wish aloud for this baby inside me to be a boy.

We're cooking dinner in the kitchen of our condo the next night when he pauses as he sautés chicken at our stove. "I thought of a story I haven't told you yet," he says with a smile, and I raise my chopping knife in the air and praise the Lord for the gift I am about to receive from his bounty, amen.

"Tell me now," I say. I'm roughly eight months pregnant at this point, and even if the smell of chicken and vegetables makes me want to vomit, this potentially new piece of information about Aaron is all I need to survive anyway.

I take a break from preparing our salad and lean expectantly over the kitchen island, bracing my arms on either side of it.

"Aaron. Now."

He's already giggling in his most authentic way: with a shake of the shoulders that means he is already thoroughly entertained with a story he can't yet get out. He proceeds to tell me about a game he played with himself after his parents' divorce, when his mother, a young flight attendant, moved her two children out of the home she shared with her now-ex-husband and into a small two-bedroom apartment in the northern suburbs of Minneapolis. It's a far-northern suburb we're talking about, with split-level tract homes from the 1970s and tired, featureless apartment buildings lining the two-lane highway that cuts through town. There are many towns like this across America, which seem like they have always been weary and beaten, by weather and by the difficulties of the lives unfolding inside them.

Aaron was ten when his parents split up, suddenly sharing a room with his little sister. He insists the divorce was no big deal to him, that he knew from a young age it wasn't going to work out between his parents, but he also tells me that he and his sister never slept in their bedroom, that Nicole and their mother would spend the night in their mother's bed, Aaron curled up in a sleeping bag on the floor beside them. Not because he was scared, he says, he just liked the feeling of the three of them being close. A unit. A team.

What Aaron wants to tell me about is a game, a game that to a woman who took not one but *two* psychology courses in college clearly illustrates how not-traumatic his parents' divorce was. He played it when visiting his friends, and, um, he would rank his friends on how likely it would be for him to be able to *live in their bathrooms*? All kids are weird, but I definitely never considered the bathrooms of my friends' homes for my primary residence, and I want to know more. It was easy, he tells me. He had criteria: Could he lay out a sleeping bag? Would there be a place to store necessities like small dishes and personal belongings? Was it warm? Comfortable?

The clear winner was a wealthier friend whose parents' master bath had both a tiled bathroom area and a carpeted dressing area with a vanity, where Aaron could imagine unfolding his sleeping bag and hunkering down for the rest of his life.

He's laughing so hard he can barely get it out, and I'm laughing so hard that the kitchen island is holding up my breathless, pregnant body. I definitely peed in my leggings. Just a little bit.

When I'm done laughing, I'm suddenly crying. Big, round tears that wash off my mascara and soak my shirt. Thick sobs that turn my face red and make my nose run. It's an emotional flash flood, and Aaron is watching from dry land, shocked and amused and horrified all at the same time and all I can say when he asks what the hell is wrong is that I don't know, but I do know.

I'm crying because I'm pregnant and crazy and totally out of control and the universe is random and there is no order to things and when I look at this man who so gracefully deals with a shitty reality he doesn't deserve I can perfectly see the little boy who imagined living in his friends' bathrooms and the poignancy and beauty of this very moment is too much for me to bear. I can never say it, I can barely even think it, but I know that I am crying because I am afraid that when Aaron is gone, there will still be parts of him I do not know, little things like this that he forgot to share with me. I'd felt that from the moment I met him, before we knew he was sick, but I feel it more urgently now: like I want to just stick a little USB drive into his arm and download everything about him. I want every memory, every feeling, every thought from baby Aaron and child Aaron and punky teenage Aaron, who pierced his ears multiple times. Grown-up Aaron hugs me close to his skinny chest until the fire alarm lets us know we've burned our dinner to the pan.

When our relationship started Aaron and I had traded these little pieces of ourselves so freely and so immediately that we both started to fear we might run out sooner than we'd anticipated, that our respective wells would run dry and we'd end up just like the couples we pitied, passing the saltshaker without even looking up from our crossword puzzles or even worse, a game of Candy Crush.

But love is funny, and there's something about the thrill of discovering another person that makes even a story you've heard before a story you want to hear again and again, like the childhood books whose spines wore out from so many bedtime readings.

I HAD A HIGH SCHOOL teacher who was obsessed with the Vietnam War. We called this teacher Bilbo Baggins, in part because he was small and beardy, and in part because all high school kids are terrible people who should be caged until they are at least twenty-one. Really, though, the joke was on us because Bilbo Baggins is a damn hero and that guy, like most high school teachers, was a saint.

"You know what I would love?" he said one day, pacing the room in his worn, wide-wale corduroys and loafers. "I'd love for a real Vietnam vet—a guy who was *your age* when he fought a *war*—to walk through this door and tell us his story." He was just talking to himself, but my good friend and one-time boyfriend Guy raised his hand and announced, "Nora's dad is a Vietnam vet!"

"Is that true?" Bilbo asked, and I nodded. What I didn't say was that my father had never talked about it, not to me, not to my siblings. What I didn't say was that his time as a marine, when he really was just a kid, was a point of quiet pride for him. That it imbued him with the fastidiousness he still carries today: A place for everything, and everything in its place. Take all you want, but eat all you take. Take the message to Garcia. *Semper Fi.* Stand up straight, goddammit.

"So," my dad says over dinner that evening, reaching across me to take seconds, "I'll see you tomorrow at school."

"What are you *talking* about?" I ask, suddenly racking my brain for any rules I may have broken that would necessitate a meeting with my parents at school. How many times did I get a uniform violation for having my shirt untucked? Is that an offense punishable by a secret parent-teacher conference?

"Your history teacher called!" he says, almost giddily. "I'm coming in to talk to your class."

I'm shocked not because my father isn't a generous man, but because he is such a private one. I've never seen the man naked—though, who wants to see their parents naked?—he wears a bathrobe over his pajamas, always, the ultimate in modesty. He called the past Christmas "total bullshit" because my mother gave me a water bra from Santa. Why Santa cared enough about my flat chest to give me a bra that simply included a set of water balloons stitched inside the cups was beyond me, but I was grateful to suddenly have a B cup underneath my school polo. Most of what I knew about my father and the life he lived before I was born, if you can call that a life, even, had come to me slowly, usually as we drove around the city that raised him.

"See that?" he'd say, pointing vaguely out the driver's-side window. "That's the tree my sister used to have me climb as a kid to steal her green apples. She'd give me a paper bag and tell me to jump the fence and fill it up."

I loved those moments, when he would give me a piece of himself without my asking, a little treasure just for me.

My dad is already in the classroom when I arrive. History is the third period of the day, right before lunch, and my typically squirrelly classmates are all seated quietly when I arrive because my dad has the kind of face that tells teens he does not fuck around. I'm sweating profusely, nervous both for my father and for myself, because even when you truly love your parents as a teenager, you are also horrified by nearly everything about them.

Nothing about my father screams "Vietnam vet!" to a group of kids whose main Vietnam reference is Forrest Gump's Lieutenant Dan. My dad is one of the lucky men who arrived home physically unharmed and able to keep their emotional wounds from seeping through to the surface, though sometimes at night I will hear him cry out in his sleep from down the hall. He looks like any other middle-aged white guy, really: gently parted hair, polo shirt, khakis. Just any old Bill O'Reilly fan who has taken a break from his daily golf game to stand in front of a few dozen teenagers at his alma mater and tell them the dark things he hasn't spoken about in decades.

It's silent for the full fifty minutes while my father talks, and I'm surprised by the fact that he's prepared transparencies of the country of Vietnam for the overhead projector and by the fact that when he begins, I can sense a small tremor in his voice. Nothing anyone else would notice, just a small signal in a frequency detectable only by those who love you.

My father's only mementos from the war are a sweatshirt so small that I've worn it since I was twelve, when it was the closest thing to a grungy-skater-girl outfit I could muster when my parents wouldn't let me shop at Urban Outfitters, and a small shadow box with a few snapshots, his bars, and a swastika pendant—an auspicious symbol in Buddhist cultures, a gift from a villager. As I watched, during those fifty minutes, that entire shadow box came alive. I saw my father, in his late fifties by then, as the eighteen-year-old who left these same classrooms to ship himself off to war as an enlisted marine. He was just a boy when he carried these dead friends on his back. This is the first I've heard of any of these boys, these ghosts he has carried with him for over thirty years.

When he is done speaking, he offers to answer any questions from the class, and my entire body tenses.

"What's the worst thing that happened to you?" this dipshit

named Mark with a butt cut asks my father, and I feel every hair on the back of my neck bristle. The fuck's the matter with this kid—besides his haircut and his Uncle Fester face—that he would ask my father this question, clearly so off limits in so many ways?

But my father doesn't skip a beat. He tells us about struggling to pull the body of a fallen marine onto a helicopter during heavy fire, how one of his friends stepped forward to help and was instantly killed by a bullet that would have instead ripped through my father's own skull.

Mark lowers his head, unable to meet my father's earnest gaze. The bell rings, but nobody stands up until my father dismisses them.

After class, I follow him out into a bright, hopeful Minnesota afternoon to play hooky for a daddy-daughter lunch. I don't ask him about anything he just told me and a bunch of other teenagers; I just settle into the passenger side of his black Lincoln with all his ghosts.

JUST A FEW MONTHS AFTER their deaths I struggle to recall the details of these favorite tales from my husband and my father. Was it when he was nine or ten when a strange boy at the playground asked to see Aaron's basketball, then kicked it across the highway? How possible is it that I could find that boy today, now an adult male close to forty, and kick his ass? What was my father's company, again? First Battalion, Alpha Company? First Recon Division? The Hawks? No, that's a sports team. No, it's an animal.

Today I went to another funeral. As a Catholic, funerals are both ritual and social engagement. Today's funeral was for a high school friend, a man my age named Eddie, married just a month ago, who died of the cancer that killed Aaron. The Basilica is *the* basilica, the first in our country, an imposing Beaux Arts building just under the freeway, on the edge of downtown Minneapolis. In its one hundred years the Basilica has seen many thousands of graduates and brides and baptized babies. Fifteen years ago, the class of 2001 lined up in these pews, in front of a massive marble altar, under the open arms of the Virgin Mary, and officially matriculated into adulthood. Now we are here to bury our classmate, and I cannot begin to list all the ways that this is not okay.

The day was two parts funeral, one part high school reunion, so I was glad to arrive at the Basilica of Saint Mary with cystic acne and baby boogers on the shoulder of my J.Crew swing coat to really show my high school classmates I was doing a-okay, even if I didn't live up to being voted Most Likely to Have a Talk Show. Also, I'd like to see the statistics on how many people did live up to what they were voted to be in their senior yearbooks. Although our Most Likely to Succeed is a dentist, so good for her/why am I such a failure?

We all remember differently, and that may never be more apparent than when you see people you haven't seen in over a decade. It is obvious, standing with a group of cute high school boys who grew into handsome men, that the truth is a multifaceted object, that it is slippery and subjective. Zach remembers me as pretty, his ultimate crush, and I am simultaneously flattered and totally incredulous because I remember spending all of high school convinced that I was the ugliest person alive. I think the polite and appropriate thing to do when someone is effusing over your past beauty is just to nod and give a sincere thank-you. But if you're wondering how joking that "hey, I'm single now" would go over in a church, after a funeral, in front of people you haven't seen for over a decade, four months after your husband's death, let me just save you the trouble and say . . . not great? Work on the punch line and revisit it in a few months.

After I killed the vibe at a funeral, my classmates and I joined everyone else in the massive church basement for lunch. This basement is filled with so many people that I do not know: people who Eddie went to college and school with. His cousins and his coworkers. We all lead many lives that rarely intersect. It's so uncomfortable for me, watching another person's worlds mix together; I can't imagine how I'll feel watching my own funeral as a really beautiful ghost.

People are uncomfortable with the idea of a microphone, and it's been a slow trickle of those brave enough to stand up and tell a story, when Eddie's cousin takes the mic.

"Please," he says, "if you knew Eddie in a different way than I did, tell me a story now." He is soft and ruddy-cheeked, with small eyes made smaller by crying. "Tell me anything," he says, before sitting back down to lunch. "Give me a way to hold on to him." I had said almost the same thing to a group of friends after Aaron died, when all my memories of him were occluded by the horror of the past month. "Help me remember him," I texted, and they filled my phone with funny photos and stories until he came back to me as he'd lived, not as he'd died.

I want this for Eddie's cousin, though I am too embarrassed to stand and speak. I want to tell him about how Eddie got drunk on prom night, in the block of hotel rooms our friend's parents had rented for all of us, because we were such good kids and probably, a little bit, because their daughter had fought serious complications from cystic fibrosis her whole young life and deserved to have a dream prom, complete with an unsupervised post-prom party. We'd all ditched our expensive dresses for basketball shorts and sweatshirts and sometime in the middle of the night (or, more realistically, about 11:00 P.M.), Eddie stumbled drunk into the room where I was Frenching my boyfriend and decided my prom dress must be the bathroom. That memory tended to get lost somewhere for me, pushed out by trivia from the *Real Housewives* franchise and too many tweets, but Eddie brought it up every time I saw him over the years.

"Remember when I peed on your prom dress?" he'd say, laughing like it was just yesterday that I had to point his drunk teenage ass toward the actual bathroom while wringing out my prom dress into a hotel trash can.

I will never forget that story again, and I will need to dry-clean that dress before my imaginary daughter wears it to Prom 2032.

AARON AND MY FATHER HAVE been gone for months now, and it hurts in a different way than it did at first. I feel sometimes like an archaeologist, discovering new ways to miss someone as I discover new things about them.

In Aaron's wallet, I find a small Post-it note, something I'd left behind on the counter as I left for work, right when he'd first started treatment.

> *Feel better. I love you. So much.*
> *Love,*
>   *Nornia*

Of all the notes I left him, this one made it front and center in his wallet, in front of all his credit cards. I will never know why this one was so special to him, but it is enough to know that it *was* special, that I did small things that meant a great deal to him, the way he did for me.

I did my best to memorize Aaron and my father, to know them by heart the way I knew my beloved childhood books, which I could recite from memory even when full pages went missing, but it was an impossible task. I know they will continue to come to me like this, in unexpected notes and memories, helping me to fill in the missing pages.

Chapter 4

Brothers Gotta Hug

My siblings and I often communicate in nothing but movie lines. The sophisticated and mature all know that you can convey a lot of emotions through the scripts of *Tommy Boy, Black Sheep, Dumb & Dumber,* and *Stepbrothers.*

I was just checking the specs on the endline for the rotary girder . . .

I know you just caught me Googling "burial at sea" when I was supposed to be looking up directions to the funeral home.

Just when I thought you couldn't get any stupider . . .

Could you not buy my two-year-old a singing plastic hamster?

You gave our dead bird to a blind kid?

You know you're an idiot, right?

Brothers don't shake hands, brothers gotta hug!

I know you're really scared and sad about your husband dying, but I am here for you. And I will still try to make you laugh until you pee your pants.

Having three siblings does have its downsides, like when you have explosive diarrhea and your sister is in the bathroom working on her bangs or your brother breaks your tailbone while you're wrestling for the remote control and you get sent to your room because you said the f-word. But there are upsides, too. Like having three best friends to take care of you while your husband enters hospice a few weeks after you all lost your father.

I expected that of Meghan, because Meghan has been like a mom to me. She's eight years older, which doesn't make her actually old enough to be my mother, but in the eighties it was totally socially acceptable for her to assume primary responsibility for me while our parents were busy. And she did a good job except for the time I launched my baby walker down the concrete steps while she was flirting with our neighbor boy.

As the oldest child, Meghan blazed the trail for all of us, but especially me. She was the first child to move out (at seventeen, with a full-time job and her own apartment). The first to get a tattoo, dye her hair pink, publish a book, get married, have a child, and become a notable figure in the Minneapolis business community. I'm basically a knockoff version of Meghan, in many ways. But I am taller.

Meghan was the first person I called when we knew the baby inside me was dead. I didn't need to say anything: she knew everything from the way I said her name. She picked me up early the next morning, sat with me in the waiting room with our sister-in-law, held my hand until they took me away to scrape the baby out of me. When I woke up, in a druggy haze, I told her I wanted to go to the mall to buy new panties. I'd always hated that word, but I kept saying it, kept insisting that I needed new panties, that we must go to the mall to buy new panties. "Okay," she said, as the nurse shook her head and silently mouthed the word *no*. At home, she tucked me into bed next to Aaron and handed me my credit card, where I promptly ordered thirty new pairs of underpants because a quasi-abortion really puts you in a weird head space. "I love you, Nor Nors," she said, kissing me like I was her own child. She was there when Aaron was in hospice, perpetually cleaning my kitchen, raising my child, and giving me healthy pours of white wine to anesthetize me at night.

I expected a lot of Patrick, too. He's the youngest, and just two years younger than me, so I consider him "my" brother. We were raised as a pair, like Austin and Meghan were. Patrick has all the idiosyncrasies of an elderly man in a twenty-nine-year-old body. He "collects" cars, by which I mean his driveway is filled with automobiles in various states of functionality. He "is getting really into clocks." He's "got a guy," whether you need a vintage refrigerator door or a new deck built. His quirks are not studied and affected. Rather, they are the kind of genuine weirdnesses that eventually end up in the pages of Urban Outfitters catalogs. Things like handlebar mustaches and old cassette tapes and man buns. He is the kind of man who has an ironic tattoo inside his upper lip, and also spends a lot of his time on recreational birding.

Patrick and Aaron shared a special bond. They loved comic books and superhero movies and making fun of me for having lived in New York. "Oh!" they'd say to each other. "Did you know that Nora used to live in *New York*?! I mean, *wow*." I'd always wanted the man I loved to love my family the way I do. Aaron and Patrick loved each other perhaps more than either of them loved me, and I was okay with that.

But I had basically no expectations of my brother Austin. Austin is seven years older than me, and he was always Meghan's brother. Whereas a much older sister will mother you, a much older brother will ask you to please stop coming down to the basement and interrupting his Dungeons & Dragons game or he'll fart on your head.

My father always insisted that Austin was our mother's favorite child, because he most closely resembles her. I think he is her favorite because he is a cipher. He doesn't give much away, you have to draw it out of him, or just search through his dresser drawers while he's at school. He is quiet and contemplative, right-handed, and has an Ivy League degree. Which in a family of loud, obnoxious lefties makes you a total black sheep.

Austin's slipperiness just made me more intrigued by him, and I followed him around like something that is more annoying than a puppy, while he swatted me away for years and years. For a few years when we were both on the East Coast, we'd visit each other by train and spend the weekends smoking pot and watching *It's Always Sunny,* and every time I made him laugh I would think to myself, *My cool brother finally loves me!!!* while outwardly trying to play it cool. But when he moved to Seattle, the years and distance pulled us apart again.

The night that Aaron entered hospice, Austin came to our house and spent the night on my couch, away from his own wife and child. He took a leave from work and spent every day just being there. Austin had just moved back to Minneapolis, and he and Aaron had barely gotten to know each other, but he showed up. Like, really showed up, which is more important than just physically being there. It is hard to die with dignity, because the dying process does everything it can to strip you of it, day by day. I did what I could do myself, but I needed help, and Aaron knew it. Who was okay to see him like this, I asked, who could help me do these very personal things? "Just you and my brothers," he told me in his fading, scratchy voice. Patrick and Aaron had called each other "brother" since the day they met, but Austin became Aaron's brother when it mattered most. And both of them made sure that Aaron died as well as he could, wearing a button-down shirt because he liked to look like a damn gentleman.

Patrick read comic books aloud to Aaron, and Austin sat with him for hours in the room that was our office, holding his hands. My slippery brother was there, every day. No longer a mystery to me, but a constant reassurance in the face of death and loss. When I woke up, he was in my kitchen. When I went to bed, I heard him saying good night to Aaron. "It's okay, buddy," he told him, "I'll take care of them. You did good. You did real good."

We learn as we get older to appreciate the people we love for who they are, and for how they love us. I realized that my dad was never going to be Danny Tanner, and I loved him for the way he *could* love me, which was sometimes a little too sarcastic for a child to understand. My mother is not my best friend, but I can appreciate her own unique brand of love, even if I sometimes want to kill her. Patrick and Meghan always loved me the way I love them: out loud and aggressively. It is completely normal for us to get into screaming fights, or laugh until we pee our pants. Sometimes at the same family dinner.

Austin will always be quiet and contemplative, and his love for us will always be a steady and reliable force even when the floor gives way beneath us. But maybe it has always been this way. My mother loved to tell us how Austin would come home from school when I was a baby, creep into my nursery, and carry me downstairs, claiming I'd already been awake, to have a chance to play with me. And wasn't it Austin who told me to study abroad during college, to not be afraid of leaving behind my boyfriend and exploring the world? Maybe that was actually my dad, but I do remember Austin running to a neighbor's house to get a pair of scissors when my shoelaces got caught in my bike gears, which meant at one point, he had taken his little sister out for a bike ride. Because he did like me, at least a little bit. And he maybe even loved me, in his own quiet way, while I was just too damn loud and obnoxious to hear it.

I don't have to chase Austin around anymore, I know. He's going to be there for me for the rest of my life, whenever I need him, as long as I promise never to go through his drawers again. In the immortal words of John C. Reilly and Will Ferrell in the critically acclaimed, Oscar-winning movie *Stepbrothers:*

"Did we just become best friends?"

"Yup!"

Chapter 5

Take the Message to Garcia

S teve had high expectations for his four children. And why wouldn't he? Before he'd even turned twenty-one, he'd spent several years as a marine, served in a war, and become an accomplished alcoholic.

"Stand up straight," he'd bark, slapping me on the back just between my shoulder blades. "Roll those shoulders back and put them in their pockets!" I cannot imagine that last part being a marine phrase, but I repeat it to every sloucher I see because poor posture really is such an unattractive trait.

In addition to disapproving of bad posture, Steve wasn't much for excuses, either.

"You need to take the message to Garcia," he'd insist when we offered up reasons for not returning our rental videos on time, for not mowing the lawn or unloading the dishwasher or completing our homework.

"What does that even *mean*?" we would whine, as he thrust a plastic bag into our hands and pushed us out the door toward the piles of dog shit that had accumulated in the yard while we were too busy "studying" to clean up after the dog we'd sworn we'd take care of.

"It *means,*" he said, "that when something needs to be done, you goddamn do it!"

That's another marine/Dad thing, I think, placing swears in awkward places where they don't exist.

No matter what our excuses were, my father's answer was always the same.

"My bike tires are out of air, so I can't bike to work."
"Take the message to Garcia."

"I got a C because my teacher hates me."
"Take the message to Garcia."

"I think my arm is broken."
"Take the message to Garcia."

My siblings and I still love this phrase, even if we were never really sure where it came from. Not because my dad didn't explain its origins, but because he explained it to us so many times that we just took for granted that he'd always be there to try to drill a life lesson into us.

Here's the CliffsNotes version. And by CliffsNotes, I mean Wikipedia. So, America is about to get into a war with Spain. And President McKinley needs to get a *message* to General Garcia in Cuba. Because he just does, okay? Anyway, McKinley is sitting around wondering how they're going to get this message to Garcia in Cuba, and he can't think of anyone. I kind of imagine him look-ing around at a table full of guys who are just avoiding eye contact and hoping they don't get called on, until his eyes meet with a young guy named Lieutenant Rowan and it becomes immediately obvious: This is the guy. He will take the message to Garcia. I know this isn't how it actually happened, history buffs. Just relax, I'm telling a story and using Wikipedia in place of my dad, okay?

So Rowan takes the message to Garcia. That's the whole point. He doesn't ask, as my dad pointed out to me every time I tried to claim I didn't know how to start the lawn mower, *how* to get there. He didn't ask *why* he had to take the message.

This is kind of a heavy concept to get through your thick skull when you are young and stupid and just want to watch MTV and paint your nails, but dammnnnnnnn, Steve had a good point, because I have a bad habit of not taking the message to Garcia, but instead saving the message to Garcia as a draft and forgetting about it for seven to ten days or weeks. And I have my ~~excuses~~ reasons.

For one, I am really tired. I didn't get a ton of sleep last night because I was up too late binge-watching *Orange Is the New Black*. Also, my phone died and I recently lost all my contacts and some-thing came up at the last minute and I didn't have a baby-sitter so I couldn't make it, sorry. Also, I just lost two hours of my life going down an Instagram rabbit hole and now I'm following a guy who has spent $100K to make his face somewhat resemble a drawing of Kim Kardashian and I'm 99 percent sure I should probably get a nose job, right? Also, I was on Google last night and then I ended up on WebMD diagnosing myself with a rare cancer, so I probably shouldn't plan on taking any messages to anyone, at least not until my treatment is over.

I don't have my dad to remind me of Rowan anymore, so I have to remind myself to take the message to Garcia. I hate that, because I miss my dad and also because I am lazy. I don't *want* to learn how our furnace works and why it is broken. It was Aaron's job to set up the Apple TV and troubleshoot all my tech issues, not mine. I bought the bike trailer for Aaron to use with Ralph, but now it's my job to make sure our son tools around our city with a good view of my butt. I am not an incredibly confident driver, but it turns out I can load up and drive a moving truck on my own. And every time I cross something off my to-do list that wouldn't be there if my husband or father were still alive, I feel perhaps prouder than I should for just being an adult. It is annoyingly true, as we find out once we try to have our tattoos removed or find out the boyfriend our mothers never warmed up to is moving out east to join a "throuple," that our parents are sometimes right. My excuses usually *are* stupid. I'm more capable than I think I am and no, I probably don't have a rare form of cancer.

I can take the message to Garcia. It doesn't matter how or why. When something needs to be done, I can goddamn do it.

Chapter 6

Where Is My Syllabus?

Most people in college skipped the first day of class.

"It's just syllabus day," my friends said, laying in their twin beds, playing Snood on their Dell laptops, "it's not like you're going to miss anything."

"I know, so dumb," I agreed, my backpack on nice and tight, because nobody in Minneapolis had bothered to tell me what the hell Vera Bradley was, let alone buy me a loud, quilted bag that looked like one an old lady would hide her knitting in.

Then I hightailed it across campus with my signature speed walk. Because also nobody had bothered to tell me that it was cooler to walk slow than it was to shout, "On your left!" while zipping around people on the paths that crisscrossed our tiny campus.

I wasn't about to miss my favorite day of the semester.

I had a routine for syllabus day. I'd arrive to class early, choose a seat near the front but not quite in the front row, and crack open my Franklin Covey planner and a fresh notebook, scrawling my name across the top page like I had since I learned to write in cursive: *Nora Elizabeth McInerny.*

Why would you want to miss this day, where the teacher would hand you a literal roadmap to success—the exact steps you needed to take to get an A, stay on the dean's list, and earn your father's respect and admiration—printed on a few sheets of 8½-by-11-inch paper? We'd go through the syllabus as a class, walking through each of the items, which as biological adults we should have been able to read over on our own time. No matter, each teacher was happy to expound on the upcoming reading assignments and their expectations for research papers and essays.

"Questions?" the professor would ask, and I'd shake my head, copying each upcoming assignment into my planner, with a reminder the week before that a due date was approaching. It didn't matter how drunk I got at Soupie's bar using the expired driver's license of my friend's ex-boyfriend's older sister, a thirty-year-old named Melanie Beaulieu who was a five-foot-six, 110-pound Sagittarius from De Peres, Missouri. Those assignments were getting done. I was getting an A.

I'd been getting A's since it was possible to get an A, and I'd have done it sooner if my grade school hadn't offered up ridiculous options like U (unsatisfactory), S (satisfactory), or the covetable S+ (more than satisfactory). I'd pore over my report cards each quarter, relishing the comments from my teachers, hellbent on turning any S into an S+ the next time that yellow sheet of paper showed up on the dining room table.

When I crossed the stage at the Xavier University Cintas Center in May 2005, it was with a hangover and a BA in English, magna cum laude.

"Why not summa?" my dad asked, and I flushed with shame, remembering the Latin class I'd had to drop my freshman year when it became apparent that learning a dead language just wasn't in my wheelhouse if I wanted to keep up my aggressive drinking schedule.

Like our graduation speaker told us, our whole lives stretched ahead of us, an awesome sea of possibility. What she didn't tell us—what nobody was telling me—was where the fuck I was supposed to go or do next.

I had to start my grown-up life somewhere, so the day after graduation, I dragged my hungover body out of bed and headed back home. I cried for what seemed like the entire twelve-hour drive from Cincinnati to Minneapolis, smoking the free cigarettes we'd been handed at the bar by a cigarette "street team" of recent graduates who had used their degrees to help recruit the next wave of lung cancer patients.

I drove my green Honda Civic, with its single-disc CD player, through the flat expanse of Ohio and Indiana for six straight hours, a printed, stapled list of directions from MapQuest as my navigator. My cell phone had been tragically killed in a drinking accident the night before, so I was in transit, incommunicado and in total crisis for most of my drive, listening to Stevie Nicks singing the lyrics of "Landslide" directly into my soul, on repeat. *Could* I sail through the changing ocean tides? *Could* I handle the seasons of my life?

The answer was a heartfelt and off-key "Ooooooooooooh, I don't know."

When you are an English major, they tell you that you can do anything, but what they really mean is that you could just as easily end up doing nothing. I was confident, reading all those books and writing all those papers, that I was being prepared for greatness, and somewhere outside of this generic Midwestern college campus was a job with my name on it. All I had to do was let the world know

I was available, and they'd be lining up for the chance to show me what was next. After all, this was the heyday of Jessica Simpson on *Newlyweds,* of Paris Hilton and *Laguna Beach.* Success, it seemed, was just a given if you were a moderately attractive white girl with blond hair and no shame.

To the credit of the entire world, who eventually lost interest in all three of those things, that was not exactly the case. The world was not waiting for another blond white girl whose interests were "I dunno, lots of things" and whose stated goal on her résumé was "to get a job with [name of company]."

I envied the friends who were so certain of their futures. The ones who graduated with a degree in marketing and went to work for GE or P&G or any other company that goes by just its initials, or graduated with degrees in biology and moved on to medical school, or with degrees in political science and moved on to law school. I bought an LSAT book, but kept falling asleep in my lawn chair every time I opened it. I considered business school, but then I realized that you needed to take a test to get in and decided the first test of business school is knowing that you need to take a test to get in, and I'd clearly failed. I still bought a GMAT book, and then realized that taking "Math for Athletes" with the entire basketball team hadn't exactly prepared me for the rigors of business school.

I didn't know what I wanted to be when I grew up. I was waiting for someone to tell me, but nobody did.

Nobody told me to move to Italy after graduation and take a lazy summer as an au pair while my classmates rushed off to jobs managing rental car franchises, in a big old hurry to be grown-ups with rent and car payments. I didn't get explicit instructions on how to move to New York City, though I hope that if I had, they would have advised me to have more than $400 in my bank account, and to maybe have a job lined up before arriving with my two suitcases and a dream, like Fievel Mousekewitz. I didn't know how to be single, and I sucked at it, but somehow that got me to Aaron, and I got to fall in love the way I once fell down the stairs at a movie theater: hard and publicly, with just a little bit of rug burn. There was no roadmap for me to follow when my phone rang and Aaron was having a seizure at work, or when the reason for the seizin' turned out to be a brain tumor, which turned out to be the gnarliest form of brain cancer there is. Aaron and I made it up as we went along: We got married, we had a baby, we traveled and went to concerts and sometimes got caught by the nurses getting a little too friendly in his hospital bed. This is not to say that I didn't have doubts, because I did. I was sure, all the time, that I was doing it wrong. I spent a lot of time looking up from my life and craning my neck around to get a glimpse at everyone else's paper: How were they adulting, and were they doing it better than me? Should I be buying a house in the Midwest instead of renting in Brooklyn? *Should* I be getting an MBA or at least marry someone who has one? Am I taking good enough care of Aaron? Is it okay that I'm still working while he's sick, even though he tells me I should? Should I maybe *not* have left my full-time job when my husband died?

I thought I was ready to say good-bye to Aaron. "It's okay," I told him, "I'll be okay." After three years of chemo and radiation, every labored breath was truly work for his body. The pain of a brain tumor was so immense that he was on a list of narcotics I'd only heard about drug addicts using, and during his two weeks of hospice he'd slipped slowly from my side into a quiet, unconscious limbo between this world and the next.

The moment he was gone, I wasn't ready anymore, and I was filled with a crippling sense of doubt. *Was I good enough for you? Did I make this easy enough? Why did I get mad at you for forgetting garbage day? What the fuck do I do now?*

At twenty-two, with an expensive degree and no plan for my life, I felt like a fucking loser.

At thirty-two, with an expensive degree, a mortgage, a child, and no plan for my life, I feel like a fucking genius.

Somewhere in those past ten years, I became, against all odds, an adult. Emails started arriving in my inbox from recent grads with dreams of working in PR and marketing, asking me what I thought they should do. My sixteen-year-old neighbor burst through my back door with her finger wrapped in a pile of bloody paper towels after slicing it open trying to halve a bagel. My response to both situations was an internal, *So, why are you talking to* me? And then it hit me: They thought I was an adult! Oh shit, I *was* an adult! I somehow bandaged up the girl next door and got her finger to stop gushing blood on my granite countertops, and I replied to nearly every email I got from younger women looking for advice. But I told them all the same thing: I have no idea what I'm doing, and it's okay if you don't, either.

I know that I will never be ready to be an adult, that nobody will ever give me the proper instructions, and even if they did, I'd treat them like I do most maps or IKEA manuals and wing it anyway. Being an adult is doing everything before you are ready. It's having the guts or blind stupidity to take your own route and make it up as you go.

I was never going to move to Cleveland and stay at home with my two children while my banker husband brought home the organic, nitrate-free bacon. I was never going to be a lawyer or an MBA, though all three of those are fine things to be.

I was always meant to find my own weird little path in life, no matter how many years I spent following the one laid out for me.

I still sometimes feel that gnawing feeling that I am doing it wrong, that I should be more like my friends with normal jobs and normal lives, but I know that the voice inside me is sometimes an idiot, because that voice is the same one that convinced me to get the Reese Witherspoon *Sweet Home Alabama* haircut even though I'm six feet tall with a weak chin and ended up looking like a brontosaurus. I don't know what is next, and that's okay. It's more than okay, because I actually get to decide what it is. I can keep inventing this life as I go, creating the world I want for myself and my son, showing him that life is best when you live it yourself, rather than waiting for someone to show you how it's done.

There is no syllabus for life that outlines the steps you need to take to graduate to the next event. This life itself is the lesson and the test and there is no dean's list and no gold stars. There is just the sum of your relationships and your actions, measured by how you feel when you lie down to go to sleep at night, and how many people heart your tweets.

I never thought I would say this, but fuck syllabus day.

Chapter 7

iPhone Therapy

I overcame myself, the sufferer;
I carried my own ashes to the mountains;
I invented a brighter flame for myself.
—FRIEDRICH NIETZSCHE

A lot of people go to therapy when their spouse dies. Or when their father dies. Or when they have a miscarriage. I don't know what other people do when all three things happen to them within a few weeks, but *I* spend ten minutes twice a day meditating with Oprah and Deepak Chopra.

I haven't paid for the full version of the app, so ten minutes is all I get. It's worth it, though, to have a little bit of time dedicated to quieting the dozen or so monkeys in my brain, wearing their fezzes and vests, clanging away with tiny cymbals.

I don't know if what I am doing is meditation or really just a guided nap, but I do it anyway, repeating the mantra endlessly in my head, using those words to suppress the urge to create a mental to-do list or run through a list of failures and embarrassments from the past thirty-two years of my life.

People don't know what to do with me. It's hard to see someone suffer, so some people don't see me at all, and some people rush to share their own personal recipes for happiness. My doorstep is filled with new packages every week: books on mourning and grief or the power of prayer. I'm given yoga passes and links to articles about "dealing with grief," like the cure for what ails me is going to be a hot take like "take your time, there is no rush."

"You know," my friends say casually, "so-and-so actually went to a therapist after her father died and she thought it really helped. . . ." And I'm sure it did help so-and-so. And it might even help me. But right now, I'm busy cobbling together my own version of therapy, which basically boils down to letting me do whatever I want, whenever I want to.

"Nora," I say, "do you want to remove that shitty tattoo you got in your twenties when you were trying to impress a roommate who didn't like you? Would you like to go to yoga in the middle of the day? Get a *new* tattoo? Maybe get some laser hair removal? Take a trip to California? Quit your stable, steady job and be a stay-at-home mom whose one child goes to day care full-time?"

The answer is a resounding "yes!" and I do it all.

I run. I do yoga. I drink a lot of wine and watch ancient seasons of *Real Housewives*, specifically the inaugural Orange County season that started it all, because I find comfort in a simpler time, when the world was all about Juicy tracksuits and Paris Hilton was our most controversial celebrity. I stay up until 2:00 A.M. reading, until Ralph unfailingly wakes up crying for me. He just wants to cuddle in Mama's bed, and his slow, steady breath lulls me to sleep. He likes sleeping in, too, so our mornings are nice and lazy. Sometimes, I drop him off at day care still in my pajamas and retainer, and curl up on the couch with coffee for an hour before I even open my laptop to work. I cancel plans with friends and acquaintances, turn inward as much as I can.

I go to Catholic mass at churches where nobody will recognize me, and I watch the faces of the faithful, elderly congregants. I want what they have: an unfailing North Star to guide them. I watch the first ten minutes of a Scientology documentary and think to myself, *All right, now I can see how this would be appealing. . . .* I am slightly jealous of all the recovering alcoholics in my life, with the steady rhythm of weekly AA meetings to keep them on the straight and narrow, eyes to God. I wonder how long it would take me to develop a drinking problem, or if I may already be there.

I am creating my own path through my own grief, toward my own version of happiness.

TO BE CLEAR, I *HAVE* been in therapy before, when I was young and my life was free of any tangible problems.

"Why are you seeing a psychiatrist?" my high school boyfriend asked me when I told him about my upcoming appointment. He was truly shocked. "Are you crazy or something?"

"I don't know," I told him, staring out the window of his father's 1985 BMW, crying. "I'm just sad all the time and I don't know why." He didn't get it, and neither did I. I was on the honor roll. I played varsity sports. I had a boyfriend who was on the football team, loving parents who had been married for years. My mother bought a lime green VW Bug and I got to drive it to school every day, like Private School Barbie. But I was consumed by anxieties.

"I just feel like I could be doing more with my life," reads a diary entry of mine. "Be more successful. Be a better writer. Save more money."

I wrote that when I was ten.

I wore a pink linen maxi skirt and a white spaghetti-strap tank to my first appointment with a therapist in downtown Minneapolis. I'd scheduled it for the morning so I could still make it to my job as a lifeguard at the public pool, which opened at noon sharp. My pale Irish skin was tanned to a deep brown. "That's thanks to me and *my* people," my father told me every summer, comparing our forearms to one another. "Your mother is the kind of Irish that just burns. But not us."

I remember nothing about that appointment, not the name of my doctor or the outcome of our relationship, just the image of myself in the shiny buildings of downtown Minneapolis, my deep summer tan against my sun-bleached hair, as beautiful as I would ever be in my life, and just as sad.

"You're fucking *crazy*," my boyfriend would tell me every time we fought, and in a way, he was right. I was impatient and mercurial. I did cool things like tossing eggs and toilet paper at a girl's house because she was also dating him, and going to the MAC counter at Dayton's before a high school dance and telling the makeup artist to give me a face like Christina Aguilera. He did cool things like secretly dating girls from other high schools and calling me crazy, and I did even cooler things like hacking into his email to make sure he wasn't exchanging any secret messages with girls who weren't me and wondering why he thought I was so nuts. Incidentally, he *was* secretly messaging and dating other girls, though it is my duty to tell any teenage girls that you shouldn't read your boyfriend's private emails because it is 1) illegal and 2) I guess wrong to do.

I FOUND MY SECOND THERAPIST in my late twenties, when I had a new boyfriend whose email password was also very easy to guess

and who tried to tell me that his membership to a secret message board for New York massage parlors that were really "massage parlors" wasn't what I thought it was. I was one of the only
people I knew who wasn't seeing a therapist, and I didn't want to
miss out on the chance to have a full hour every other week to talk
about myself with a stranger. Plus, that old familiar sadness had
returned to me, bone-deep and impervious to the effects of drugs
or alcohol.

I was a PR girl at the time, a profession whose pressures are
matched only by those of neurosurgeons and fighter pilots, and
maybe not even by them because I've never heard of a neurosur-
geon who was found weeping on a bathroom floor over a botched
delivery of shampoo samples to a beauty magazine or literally flipping a table over at a party after drunkenly cry-dancing to "Girls
Just Wanna Have Fun." My job required me to have a BlackBerry
for all work emails, which was never to be switched off nor more
than five feet from my body at any time. Its humming was constant,
always a new email to attend to, a new "fire" to put out involving a
missed typo in a press release that nobody outside our office or our
clients' would ever read. I developed a Pavlovian response to this
new-age torture device, my heart rate elevating at anything my
body thought might be my BlackBerry alert. When RIM, the mak-
ers of BlackBerry, were crushed by the Apple iPhone, I felt more
than a twinge of schadenfreude.

My second therapist was blocks from my office, the most important (only) criteria in my selection process because I was always at
work. Her office was in the front room of a garden-level apartment
where she lived with her adult daughter. We had no chemistry,
which disappointed me. I wanted her to love me, or at least like
me, but she sat in front of me blankly and I found I couldn't artic-
ulate what exactly was wrong. Looking back, it was everything and

nothing all at once. I had a good job where I made a lot of money working on things that were of no real consequence to the world at large. I was in a relationship with a boy who was chronologically supposed to be a man by now: a thirty-year-old with a passion for pot and a lot of big dreams that poured out of his mouth like smoke and disappeared just as quickly.

I had high highs because I had a lot of access to really good pot and unlocked Brooklyn rooftops, and I had low lows because I had a really stressful job and nothing resembling any sort of purpose.

She wrote me some prescriptions and when my mother came to visit, I told her I was crazy and depressed and had to take drugs and she said, "Okay." That week I threw them all away, but not because I felt better or worse.

"HOW DO YOU STAY HAPPY and positive?" people ask me. And I mean, they ask me this all the time. They ask me because they are going through big life things like husbands with brain tumors and they ask me because they are going through little life things and still cannot feel a spark of happiness inside. They ask me because if you look at my Instagram photos or take me to brunch, I seem to be doing okay, all things considered. I shower (a few times a week, at least), I put on lipstick (CoverGirl, preferably). I smile.

I don't know what to tell them, so I try to tell them an abridged version of my story. That I was not always like this, that I learned it from watching Aaron. His happiness was innate, but mine is not. Mine is a choice that I make, a garden that I tend to every single day. And if you've ever seen my yard, you know that I'm a really shitty gardener, so what I am trying to say is, this is work. I do not wake up like this.

Some people have real and serious problems and should absolutely see a medical professional and maybe even take drugs.

And maybe I should, but really, I think that I spent twenty-eight years as a person who didn't know how to live, who didn't know that happiness isn't something that is handed to you, but something you have a hand in making, every day. It is harder than just getting up and grinding beans and brewing coffee, but it is just as ritualistic. For me, at least. And I don't mean this in that bullshit social media way, where people love to post little memes about how happiness is a choice, like the natural way to cure depression is to just . . . not be depressed? Because it isn't. But I'm not depressed. I'm sad. I'm in pain.

It has been four months since Aaron died. I know that this pain is temporary, but I am not in a rush to get through it. I have a friend who lost her brother and father within six months of each other, one very suddenly and one very slowly, each a jarring loss in its own way. It's been years since she buried them both, but she sends me an email one night, when the pain in my heart is razor sharp, to tell me that it will dull in time. She acknowledges that I know this, but do I know that I might miss it someday? This pain signifies how close my father and Aaron still are, and as time passes, it will bring me further away from this sorrow, but also from the two of them. Their voices will be harder to recall, their presences harder to conjure in my imagination.

At lunch with a friend recently, I find myself crying for no real reason other than the sun is shining and he is so very alive, the way that Aaron used to be. "You know," he says after hugging me, "what you're feeling is real pain. And that's not a bad thing."

There's a school of thought around this, I find out (shout out to Google for giving me a PhD in Everything). There is clean pain, what actually happens to you (e.g., your husband dies, tragically) and then there is the dirty pain, the kind you give yourself. The negative feelings (I'm a terrible person, why didn't I die?), the projections (I'm going to die alone), the anxiety around any topic at all (Should I drive in the snow? I might crash the car and die). I've lived a life, I realize, of dirty pain. Of hating myself and my body for no real reason. Of obsession and anxiety, of guilt over not living my one precious life to the fullest, whatever the fuck that even means. Aaron released me from that little self-imposed, self-conscious jail cell. He let me be myself, and he loved me even though I never fully put the cap back on anything when I'm done using it.

In many ways, my grief has been very public, but this pain, this clean pain, is mine. I don't Instagram it or blog about it or tweet about it. I keep it for myself, for late nights in bed after a bottle of wine. For moments alone in the car, driving past the homes I shared with Aaron. For throwing my keys on the counter and knowing there's no reason to call out, "We're home!" I want to keep my hand on this fire, because someday it will burn out, and all I will have to remember it by are these scars.

I have buried the two most important men in my life. I have lost a pregnancy. I have had the riptides of grief pull me out from shore in rapid succession, but for the first time in my life, I am not drowning in it.

I know that I can do it, that Aaron and my father gave me the tools I needed to live life without them. And if I need them, Oprah and Deepak are in my iPhone, waiting for me.

Chapter 8

My Eighties-Sitcom Dad

My parents referred to their brand of child rearing as Benign Neglect. I don't think that they coined the phrase, but they at least perfected it.

When my older brother was nine, he fell on his arm during a game he had invented where he jumped from a folding chair to the clothesline. Before each jump, he would move the chair back a few more inches, making his lonely game just a little more daring. I remember watching him writhe in pain on the grass while my parents went about their business. Austin was, as my father put it, a malingerer, always trying to claim some sort of disability to get out of things like going to school or setting the table. It was clear, as he turned a pale shade of green while lying on the sofa, that he was faking it. "Here," my mother said to him, rubbing some Bengay on his swollen arm, "if it still hurts after Dad is done grilling the steaks, we'll take you to the hospital." Later that night, the emergency room doctor explained to my father that kids' bones break like green twigs, staying somewhat intact even though the bone bends in on itself, not like adult bones, which snap apart like dry sticks. He also noted that my sister was relieved to hear about Austin's arm, because if they drove all the way downtown and his arm *wasn't* broken, our dad was "going to break it for him." My father assured the doctor that Meghan was autistic.

I'm not going to say that my parents fat-shamed my sister, because that term didn't exist in the eighties, but they definitely offered to pay her if she "wanted" to lose weight. When she was thirteen.

None of this sounds great, so I need to be clear that we had wonderful parents who loved each other and us, and always treated us well, even if our dad's default threat when we misbehaved was that he would "give us something to cry about."

Our parents were just . . . complicated.

Before our dad was a recovering alcoholic and writer of infomercials responsible for the clutter in your basement, he was just an alcoholic. And before that, he was a teenager in Vietnam. He was never the dad I longed for as a child, which is to say that he was not Danny Tanner. I wasn't even allowed to watch *Full House,* but I snuck enough afternoon reruns to know in my heart that I wanted the kind of dad who would respond to my emotional outbursts by sitting with me on the edge of the bed and asking me about my feelings.

Instead, I got the kind of dad who told his skinny fourteen-year-old daughter that she looked like a praying mantis. "It's not a bad thing," he said when I burst into tears. "It's just your arms and hands are freakishly long!"

Our mother also worked in advertising. She wasn't like other mothers at school, and I both loved and hated that about her. When she lost an earring—and she always lost one earring—she'd just wear the one she had, like some sort of new-wave pirate. She wore a button on her denim jacket that just read BALLS. The backseat of her car was littered with dirty coffee mugs, rolling around on the floor. She didn't hang out at school or make friends with other moms. Her friends were the collection of advertising weirdos she'd met through work: guys with Pez collections who let me play with X-ACTO knives and foam core when I came into the office with her on weekends, women who rode Harleys and helped me use the printer and binder to give my school reports a professional edge.

As long as there was money for it, she let us do absolutely every activity we wanted. She just didn't remember to pick us up from it. "Sorry!" she'd call out the window, roaring into the parking lot outside of the pool in the Geo Prizm onto which she'd let my brother caulk a plastic turtle, like a thrift store hood ornament. I'd be waiting so long after swim practice that they'd closed the pool, and my hair would freeze into little icicled dreadlocks. "I thought your *dad* was coming to get you!" she would shout, like she was talking about an estranged ex-husband and not the man she had woken up next to twelve hours earlier.

Somehow, my siblings and I grew up to be somewhat contributing members of society, with children of our own. Sure, our little brother claims to have "invented man buns" and wears adult Crocs in public and yes, my dad once saw me do the walk of shame from our neighbor's house on a Saturday morning, but overall, we turned out all right. We did not have the kind of parents who came to softball games or volunteered in our classrooms. My dad missed every college graduation but mine because he had scheduled golf trips already, and my mom went to London with friends instead of attending our little brother's first communion because one of those things is fun. They were total weirdos compared to other parents we knew. But they were consistent. About their weirdo traits and their love for us. We were loved, cared for, and taught by example that love is patient, kind, and often annoying.

When our dad was dying, I sat on the edge of his bed and rubbed his feet. He wanted to talk, and I knew that this was it: I was going to get the Danny Tanner talk I'd been waiting for my entire life.

"Nora, I'm glad you're here. I have something I want to tell you."

He said this over the course of several long and labored breaths, under the respirator that fogged up over his open mouth.

I stopped rubbing his feet for a moment and leaned in, hungrily. Even my mother looked encouraged by his sudden liveliness, like he was going to reveal the whereabouts of a buried treasure.

"It's time for you to know . . ."

I waited patiently for him to catch his breath, and see just a small hint of a smile at the corners of his papery dry lips.

"Nora," he said, breathing heavily.

"You're adopted."

Chapter 9

Family

(A Story About Juggalos and Not My Actual Family, Sorry, Siblings)

My friend Kara taught me that there are no guilty pleasures in life. There is just what you love. What you love is part of who you are, and if, like Kara, you love classic country music and red lipstick and Budweiser, if you celebrate the entire Britney Spears collection and you don't care who knows it, that doesn't make you silly. That makes you awesome. There is nothing like people who love who they are, and love what they love. It's intoxicating, even when what they love is uncomfortable and hard to understand.

I once found myself at an Insane Clown Posse concert in downtown Minneapolis, because a friend of a friend had an extra ticket and thought of me: a girl whose record collection is 90 percent Bright Eyes and 10 percent Taylor Swift. All I really knew about ICP was that they were scary to me. I can't watch any kind of horror movie at all, so the idea of listening to music that is described as "horror core," includes lyrics about chopping people up with axes, and is performed by men in clown makeup does not sound like my ideal night out.

ICP fans are commonly known as Juggalos. You've probably seen them in the parking lot of rural Walmarts or on episodes of *Cops*. For shows, they sometimes wear black and white clown face paint, hair braided into little spider legs sticking out from their heads. They commonly sport the ICP logo, an ax-wielding "psychopathic clown" on their mud flaps, T-shirts, and beer coozies, and they are known for both drinking and spraying one another with Faygo soda the way I imagine Beyoncé and Jay-Z spray each other with champagne on a regular Tuesday night after Blue is in bed and they've already swum laps in their pool of money.

I didn't grow up seeing a lot of Juggalos in Minneapolis, but they always sent a little shiver down my spine when I'd spot one in a gas station in rural Minnesota on our way up north.

Yet somehow, I went to this show with an open heart, and a few glasses of white wine in me. I also went alone, which made me even more conspicuous because I was the lone Breton stripe in a sea of JNCO jeans and belly shirts reading PSYCHO BITCH, which gave me instant outfit envy. And still, standing in the lighting booth because one of the venue employees noticed me and correctly presumed I was there for anthropological reasons and not to have my J.Crew flats soaked with high-fructose corn syrup, I looked over this crowd of misfits, being sprayed with discount cola by twenty-foot clowns who danced across the stage, and felt my little heart swell with love as the crowd sang along:

Fuck you, fuck me, fuck us
Fuck Tom, fuck Mary, fuck Gus
Fuck Darius

I was okay until they started talking about fuck Celine Dion and Tom Petty because no, we as a society must draw the line somewhere, so I focused on drowning out the music and just tuning in to the experience, which was a demented carnival show with clowns wielding chainsaws and drenching a sold-out crowd using giant water guns that pulled soda from actual barrels, and a sea of smiling faces experiencing complete and total joy.

Juggalos refer to themselves as a family, and they really are, even if they're the kind of family that has experienced at least one stabbing during a holiday get-together. At most shows I go to, crowds of too-cool white kids stand staring at their cell phones or passive-aggressively shoving one another for standing too close/ being too tall and blocking someone's view of the stage. The only people who dance are the drunkest ones, and the crowd seems to roll their eyes in unison, wishing they would just *tone it down*. The ICP show was for all ages, which meant that most of the crowd was sober, the 21+ area was actually almost empty, and there were straight-up children there. It also meant that someone brought his own raccoon? Before their heroes took the stage, the crowd chanted, *"Fa-mi-ly! Fa-mi-ly!"* And I cheered along because I knew it was going to be the only lyric that I knew and also because it's hard for me to hear people chanting and not join in.

Juggalos high-fived one another and traded their signature "whoop whoop" to greet and acknowledge one another, and I just watched them like a rock-rap Jane Goodall, feeling my affection for them grow. Most parts of society nowadays are not comfortable with shirtless men in clown makeup, or women who have PSYCHO-PATH tattooed across their throats, but for this one night, all of these Juggalos had found their place in the world, and it was the exact same venue where I came to watch Explosions in the Sky and Beach House and Chromeo, and stood awkwardly in the back, hoping I wasn't blocking anyone's view by wearing heels that made me six foot three.

I loved my ICP show for the same reason we loved seeing Caitlyn Jenner on the cover of *Vanity Fair* and the same reason my neighborhood Facebook group is obsessed with the whereabouts of a total stranger who spends every afternoon dancing with a boom box on the side of a busy street: It is rare and magical when you and your world can accept and love the same version of you.

I was hopeful, watching all of those Juggalos gleefully soaking up gallons of Faygo. They'd found their place in the world, they'd found something to love that loved them back. Maybe I could, too.

Chapter 10

A Boy Is Why I Moved to New York, and a Boy Is Why I Left

I would never actually admit that to anyone, of course. I'd tell you that I moved to New York because I had always dreamed of living there, that I was going to get a job working at a magazine and live in a stylish apartment and try my hardest to make sure a handsome, single ad exec didn't fall in love with me. "Wait," you'd say, "isn't that the plot of *How to Lose a Guy in Ten Days*?" And I'd admit that it was and tell you I moved to New York because that's where my long-distance boyfriend and I agreed to move after college.

Since fifteen, I'd never not belonged to someone. I'd set my sights on Jacob on the first day of high school, when I was six feet tall and 126 pounds, twenty of which were metal braces that made my big mouth and puffy lips even bigger and puffier.

That boy, I thought, as my mother's Geo Prizm pulled in behind his father's 1985 BMW, *will be my first boyfriend.*

It was a lofty goal, given my physical appearance, but I put in the work and made it happen just fourteen months later. "I made my dreams come true!" I wrote in my diary, very impressed with myself, even though our first kiss had ended with our teeth smashing together so hard I was sure I'd chipped one. I was proud of myself for setting a goal and seeing it through. I'd spent the early weeks of spring, when the Minnesota sun warms our city to a balmy fifty degrees, laying on a towel in the backyard, shivering, but hoping for a tan. I'd sweet-talked my orthodontist into taking off my braces after just a year, promising to wear my retainer every night. I got highlights and let the bob I'd been wearing for the past twelve years or so grow out past my shoulders. I spent the summer learning how to wear makeup and scouring the racks at T.J.Maxx and Marshall's for padded bras to make it look like I'd actually developed. And then I just hung around incessantly and broke down his defenses until he had no choice but to kiss me on the front steps of my parents' house on a snowy November evening. It was Friday the thirteenth. I was the luckiest girl in the world.

We spent the next eight years or so perfecting the art of breaking each other's hearts, then reuniting and finding new ways to hurt each other. Another girl, another boy, another big fight in an age when texting didn't yet exist, so the best way to wake up soaked in regret was to leave a message on the answering machine he shared with his three roommates after slamming eight beers on a Saturday night off campus. I picked lots of fights. I liked the way it felt, casting him away and reeling him back in like some deranged fisherman. I liked it even better when he did it to me, when I could lie in my twin bed in southern Ohio, crying over a boy who had dared to kiss another girl in his lifetime, sure he'd never speak to me again.

You know the scene in *The Shawshank Redemption* where they let that really old guy out of prison after decades behind bars, and he's so mystified by the free world that he wants to kill his boss just to get back inside? That was us after every breakup, so unable to navigate the casual-hookup culture of college that we'd just flee back to each other and the safety of our long-distance prison. I mean, relationship.

At twenty-two, I was sure that no man would ever love me aside from him, but I had a small inkling, somewhere under layers of low self-esteem, that I *could,* possibly, perhaps, maybe . . . be wrong? But I hushed that little voice, packed my two suitcases, and arrived in New York City with $400 in my checking account and no job.

My dad had given me $20 for cab fare from LaGuardia, and I watched in horror as the meter passed the $20 mark and asked whether the driver took credit cards. He did not, so Jacob had to run to the cash machine in the grocery store up the street to bail me out when I arrived at our apartment on a sticky September night.

I knew when I dropped my bags in that small studio in a run-down walkup in Astoria, Queens, with a malfunctioning lock on the front door, that we had made a terrible mistake rushing into grown-up life. But we'd signed a lease, so we spent ten months devolving from lovers to friends to resentful roommates who did things like throw out muscle shirts (me) and scream because our neighborhood's power has been out for five days (him).

On a hot summer day, just before our lease was up, my best friend, Dave, and our buddy Jimmy walked over to our apartment from their place a few blocks away. I'd gathered up a few empty boxes from the supermarket on the corner, but most of my things were stuffed into garbage bags and the two suitcases I'd brought with me nearly a year ago. Jimmy and Dave and I grabbed what we could carry in our arms and I left Jacob behind, ready to start over with a new apartment with some new girls in a new borough: Brooklyn.

IT'S A TESTAMENT TO HOW lonely and isolating New York City can be that I spent some of my prettiest, coolest years browsing the Internet for human males who lived within ten miles of me and my mattress on the floor. When I found one, Graham and I agreed, immediately, to lie about how we had met, which is always a great sign that you're embarking on a healthy relationship.

For a while, we had *fun*. We went to every show in Brooklyn, we smoked pot and drank 40s on his rooftop every night. He painted a big white square on the side of a neighboring building, and his rooftop became a movie theater just for us. But while I had to wake up every morning at seven and go to an office and climb the corporate ladder, he had a more relaxed lifestyle and work ethic. Like, maybe he'd work. Or maybe he wouldn't.

To be perfectly fair about my relationship with Graham, I was a really good girlfriend to him. I was moody and wanted him to read my mind. I loved getting too drunk and causing scenes in the hope that, like the plot of many music videos I watched in middle school, the drama would just help him realize how special I was. It would bring us closer to get in a fight in front of a taxi driver, you know? I was doing it for us. I demanded his absolute loyalty and unfailing adoration, while simultaneously seeking the approval and attention of any handsome, somewhat single male I came in contact with.

That apartment I was so proud of came with a very handsome neighbor. "Handsome" doesn't even really describe him because he was so good-looking he actually terrified me. I would see him in the hallways and suddenly find myself a mute with a plastered-on smile. Mike made sunglasses and boats in his little one-bedroom apartment, which I only knew because he once invited me in to try on some frames.

"Who's that guy I see with you sometimes?" he asked while I looked around his apartment and imagined knocking out the wall between us so we'd have room to raise our kids. I answered as honestly as I could.

"He's just a friend of mine. He's gay, actually."

I didn't break up with Graham *for* Mike—that would be insane, he had only ever said, like, three sentences to me. It's just that I knew there would be other Mikes out there, and that I needed to be with someone like him: someone with drive and ambition and a face that made me nervous to look at.

New York was making me crazy. Or crazier than normal. I started listening to *The Secret* on audiobook, and walking miles to far-off subway stations to stretch out my commute. I drank too much. I was attempting to be a vegan. At night, I would find myself with "Pop Goes the Weasel" stuck in my head for hours, thanks to the ice cream truck that parked itself outside my apartment playing a tinny instrumental version of the song on repeat, beckoning the nonexistent children in my neighborhood to come and get some frozen treats. I was always uncomfortable: In the winter, I'd freeze on my walk to the subway, only to peel off the sweaty layers on the crowded train. In the summer, my hair would stay damp even after I blow-dried it, just from humidity and sweat. My apartment was filled with $5 bodega umbrellas, because I was never prepared when it started raining. But I loved it, right?

We were in the middle of a massive heat wave, so Graham and I broke up in his bedroom, the only private space with air-conditioning that we had access to. "I'm leaving New York," I said, and I was surprised as he was to hear that.

The next day, he showed up at my door, contrite, holding his air conditioner in his arms.

"You deserve to be comfortable," he said. And even though I didn't deserve it, I let him install his breakup air conditioner in my bedroom so I could enjoy seven nights of Freon-fueled dreams before heading back to the Midwest.

Graham stopped by while I was packing up all my Forever 21 outfits in air-conditioned comfort. He was there to convince me to stay. He promised to be the kind of guy I deserved, which basically meant he wouldn't smoke pot all the time and instead just smoke pot some of the time and also have a goal or two that involved an adult future with marriage and children sometime before I was, like, forty-nine.

But it was too late for tempting promises like that. I was going back home, where for the price of my rent in Greenpoint I could afford to rent two apartments, with central air-conditioning and cable TV and furniture that I'd bought firsthand. A place where instead of a logical form of public transformation, we all just got in our SUVs alone and sat idling on the freeway, inching off to where we want to go. The kind of world where we stack our empty dishes on the edge of the table to make life easier for our server. Back to my people, who wear shorts when the temperature hits forty degrees and go running when it's zero. I was going to be close to lakes and forests and men who wear Red Wings boots because they actually *work*. Specifically, I was going back to my parents' house in south Minneapolis and the Laura Ashley dream room I'd designed when I was eleven.

Living with my parents was not the happy family reunion I'd been hoping for. Even the best parents tend to be terrible roommates. Before my dad started emailing me apartment listings from Craigslist, I'd crawl into bed after walking around the neighborhood smoking American Spirits, and wake up to Steve grinding coffee beans and telling me to get my ass out of bed and get to the store to buy him some half-and-half.

Living at home was the pits, but Minneapolis felt good to me. New York teaches you to be addicted to discomfort, but Minneapolis (when it isn't so cold you could die) makes it so easy to be comfortable.

One day when I went to check the mail, there was a note from the postman telling me to go to the post office to pick up a package. I found it annoying that he would leave a note when he could have just left the package, but as I found out that afternoon, he can't bring you the package when your ex-boyfriend hasn't actually paid what it costs to mail it to you.

I paid the remaining postage to bail my package out of post office jail, and went home to open it.

Graham had been texting furiously in anticipation of my reaction, so I knew the box contained a big, romantic gesture.

The contents were:

- 1 heart-wrenching mix CD

- 1 doughnut from my favorite doughnut shop
  (hello, Peter Pan Donuts on Manhattan Avenue in
  Greenpoint, Brooklyn. May you forever serve your
  community with delicious doughnuts and surly Polish
  teens behind the counter), a pulverized and dried-out
  symbol of our love.

- 1 T-shirt, which, as his note explained, he was
  returning to me because it was my favorite shirt.

I had never seen that shirt before in my life.

I texted him to say thank you, but threw it all in the trash. Okay, I took two bites of the stale doughnut first. But I was done. With Graham and with New York, though I'll always feel my stomach catch a little when I think of either of them. I still get nervous when my plane lands at LaGuardia, like I do when I think I see a boy I once loved at 10:00 A.M. on a Saturday at Target, when I haven't had time to put on my eyebrows or wash my hair. I think you always get that way when you see an old love: like your old self, the one he adored, could be right around the corner, young and happy and wild. When I come back to New York and my cab drives down the BQE, it passes all the rooftops I drank on with Graham, and all I see are the ghosts of the good times. I don't see myself overdrawing my checking account for the third time in a month, or getting caught in the rain and showing up to my first day of work so soaked that I had to wear a sweat suit from a stranger while my clothes dried on a heater. I just see us riding too-small vintage bikes through the cemetery, high and smiling, the best Easter I can remember. I see him pulling my shirt over my head and tumbling into bed beside me in his tiny bedroom, and the way he'd always whisper "beautiful" when he saw my bare skin. I see myself in silhouette, lying on the edge of Graham's roof, my head turned to watch the traffic lurching down Manhattan Avenue. When I turn to him, he laughs with his big smile, and it is my turn to get high. New York and Graham were fun to love, until loving them wasn't fun anymore, when I was tired of being broke and exhausted and having men jam their boners into me on crowded L trains. But I owe them both a big thank-you. For all the fun, for all the pot, for giving me the time and space to be who I was, even when I was kind of a shithead.

And then, for making it easy to leave. In Minnesota, I wasn't running toward or away from anything. I was just another good Midwestern girl with a savings account and a full-size sedan, spending her Sundays running around lakes and doing my own laundry. I was finding my own way through my new life, in the city that raised me. And I was on my way to Aaron.

Chapter 11

How I Met Your Father

Hi, Ralphie.

Right now you are only two, and you are incredibly selfish. You are always asking me to hold you or give you some grapes, and when I ask if you would prefer to perhaps poop in a toilet instead of having your grape-filled feces mashed against your nuts, you just tell me "no thanks," and hand me the butt wipes. You do show signs of promise, though. You have recently begun telling me that I am beautiful, most likely because I've started asking you to call me Beautiful Mother instead of mommymommymommymommy. You offer me your leftover milk after you've backwashed nearly half a peanut butter sandwich into it, and you let me know when you think I look tired (really appreciate that). In the mornings, you tell me you love me "SO MUCH!" and squeeze my face in your little palms.

While I'm not banking on your ever *not* pooping your pants, I'm assuming that someday, you will be interested in me as a person, and you will want to know how I met your father, the guy who is responsible for your oversize head, your sharp canine teeth, and your jolly disposition.

I'm hoping this is the case because I *love* "how we met" stories, and I want you to love all the things I love: R. Kelly, *Real Housewives*, and HGTV included. As a kid, I loved hearing how my own parents met: Grumpy was home from Vietnam, and Madame was invited by a mutual friend to his welcome home party at some ramshackle house near the University of Minnesota.

She'd heard of Steve McInerny before, but she'd never seen him, not until he came stumbling drunk down the stairs, six feet tall, 130 pounds, and deeply tanned from the Vietnam sun. *That,* she thought, *is the man I'm going to marry.* I made Madame tell me that story over and over, in great detail. Like all men who eventually become conservative old white guys, your grandfather was a dirty hippie when he was young. He had long hair, and reminded Madame of her favorite Beatle, George Harrison. When she first laid eyes on him, Grumpy was shirtless, wearing high-water bell bottoms because he'd gone shopping without trying on any of the clothes he bought.

I wanted a "how we met" story like Madame and Grumpy's: one my kids would want to hear over and over again.

I remember meeting your father at the art gallery that used to be your great-uncle Mike's photo studio. Uncle Mike's space always doubled as a site for family gatherings, from sweet sixteen parties to funerals and Thanksgivings, but when he retired, he handed the keys to his studio to a new generation of young creatives, who transformed it into an art gallery and invited what seemed like the entire city of Minneapolis to the opening.

I was there for the first time since my own grandma's funeral, standing in a space that used to belong to just our tribe, now swamped with hundreds of strangers. I'd thought your dad may be there, since we'd recently begun a Twitter flirtation, but I wasn't really sure what he actually looked like aside from the tiny, low-res avatar that represented him in his profile photo. I wore my man-eater outfit: shiny American Apparel leggings, oversize white tank top, leather bomber, Frye boots, and red lipstick. And then, I waited. And when I saw him from across a crowded room . . . I wasn't sure who exactly he was. Not until he burst into the circle I'd made with my cousins and held out his hand.

"You're Nora McInerny." He smiled.

I did what any girl would do in that situation: I reached into my bag and handed him the "Taylor Tells All" issue of *People* magazine. I knew from Twitter that he loved Taylor Swift, and he held the magazine close to his heart and thanked me.

"Oh," he said, "you know I'm not gay, right?"

My son, please know that nothing makes a girl think you are probably gay than telling her that you aren't when she hasn't even brought it up. Still, I took this possibly gay man up on his offer when he asked if I'd like to go out to a bar with him and his friends.

If you're a good dancer—which remains to be seen, because right now your go-to move is just to wiggle your legs like you're doing a toddler version of the Charleston no matter what song is playing—it will be because of your dad. I stood awkwardly on the dance floor of a shitty club in northeast Minneapolis, trying to avoid dancing, while your dad grabbed drinks for me and your aunt Lillian, who had grudgingly agreed to accompany me on an outing with a guy I vaguely knew from the Internet who may have been gay. From his spot at the bar, your dad smiled at me, busted out a little jig, and did a power slide on his knees across a crowded dance floor to deliver two Coors Lights to me and Lillian.

I knew when I accepted that ice-cold Silver Bullet that I had met a man I would definitely make out with.

It's a damn good story. Except it's not really the first time I met him, apparently.

If your dad were here, he'd tell you that we met years before, when he was working at the same ad agency where Madame had worked since I was in middle school. While I was home for a long weekend, I stopped by your grandma's office to say hello, and she walked me around to say hello to the colleagues of hers I'd known since I was a little girl. But she had an ulterior motive. As your father put it, she was "parading me around to any single guy she could find," like some sort of tour of Eligible Minneapolis Advertising Bachelors.

The pickings were slim. There was a short writer-type with a bad attitude, who later exchanged a lot of suggestive emails with me in spite of his actually having a girlfriend. There was a guy who looked almost exactly like Frankenberry from the specialty Halloween cereals I enjoyed as a child, which offered many delicious memories but not a lot of sexual excitement. Aaron was not on that tour, but he was in the cube of a young account guy who had played college lacrosse and was therefore, statistically speaking, a douchebag. Your dad introduced himself in spite of the fact that my mother considered him "kind of a goofball," which I don't remember at all, but he never forgot.

As much as I want to remember that story—especially the part where your father pined over me for *years* and followed me on Facebook and Twitter until we met again—I just don't.

We got married just a few yards away from the spot where we met—the time I remember meeting him—in that same art gallery. I point it out to you every time we drive by it. I never get sick of this story.

Love,
Beautiful Mother

Chapter 12

Please Let Me Get What I Want

A s far as first dates go, my expectations are pretty low. That will happen after a few solid years of disappointment, dating men who were made out of anything but boyfriend material.

I actually missed my first date with Aaron because of a funeral, so I'd already established myself as a hot commodity with a banging social life. And then he asked me out again. On Gchat. At the time, Snapchat didn't yet exist, so this was basically the bottom rung of the communications hierarchy. I was not impressed.

NOVEMBER 2, 2010

aaronpurmort:
wait am i allowed to ask you to hang out
over IM or are gentlemen supposed to call?

me:
i think you're ALLOWED to but
gentleman generally acknowledge that
girls plan their lives in advance

aaronpurmort:
true.
sorry. it's new to me.

me:
that's right, i forgot to wish
you a happy 13th birthday

aaronpurmort:
exactly
well if you're not furniture shopping
or making sad mix tapes, i'd enjoy
listening to some mayer hawthorne
with you. if you ARE busy, later
in the week?

me:
what time is the show?
i'm getting my hair cut

There's nothing, and I mean nothing that tells a guy you are woman in demand like letting him know he is competing with your hairstylist for your time and attention.

"I'm not going to go," I told my sister-in-law while she blow-dried my hair. Carly has been my hairstylist since she started dating my brother in about 2007. They'd been together a few months when I booked an appointment with her, which she found a little forward but I found completely appropriate because I lack boundaries. She is a really gifted stylist, and never outwardly judged me for the stripy blond "highlights" I got from the cheap Russian salon near my apartment in Brooklyn, where they charged per highlight and left me with a visual indication of just how cheap I was. If she has any flaws at all, it is that she rips through my hair with a brush like she's hellbent on punishing me for the time I called my little brother "Fatrick" when he was going through puberty and had little boy boobs.

In between punishing strokes of her paddle brush, Carly paused to make emphatic eye contact with me in the mirror.

"You're not canceling a date when your hair looks this good," she said. I hate when other people are right, but she had a solid point, so I popped the collar on that cheap leather bomber and got into my sensible Honda Accord and drove to the University of Minnesota campus to meet him for dinner at an old pharmacy that had been converted into a restaurant. He was already there when I arrived exactly eight minutes late after sitting in my car for a few minutes so as not to be the first to arrive, and he stood up to give me a hug. He smelled like . . . Old Spice and Aveda and clean laundry. And also pasta? But that might just have been the atmosphere.

He was sitting at a table, not at the bar, which meant that we were going to eat a meal. On a date. Most recently, a "date" had come to mean "grabbing a few drinks before being pawed at by an underemployed, overserved idiot," so frankly, I was a bit taken aback. I tried not to show my cards, sitting down like I was the kind of woman who routinely ate meals in restaurants and didn't subsist on late-night bowls of cereal to "soak up" the couple of beers and cigarettes she'd had for dinner.

Aaron had already ordered a bottle of wine, and the warmth of a little buzz helped calm those butterflies in my stomach until they just drifted about lazily inside of me.

"I'm just going to say it right now," he said after our entrées arrived, "when we get married, I'm going to be the stay-at-home dad."

"All right, that's fine with me," I said, because I knew from years of babysitting and lifeguarding that a career spent with children was simply not for me. I can muster enough interest in playing pretend and coloring and someone else's poop for a few hours at a time, just not as a full-time job.

Then, we just had to decide how many kids we wanted, which seemed a great topic to have over entrées. I said four, because that is how many my parents had and it really seems like the right balance. One is unacceptable. Two is just too lonely, especially if your only other sibling is a jackass. Three is all right, I guess. But four? Four is perfect. Four teaches you your place in the order of things. You learn to be gracious when you're on the top of the hog pile (is that just a thing my family did?) and patient when you're squished at the bottom. You learn to live with being farted on. You learn to be a part of a team.

Aaron wanted two, which, as I've outlined above, is just wrong, so we compromised at three and I made a mental note to pull the goalie and trick him into a fourth when our third hit kindergarten. That fourth child would be the light of our autumnal years, with nearly all the attention an only gets but none of the money because we'd have already spent it all on his older siblings.

We had a lot of other great things in common. Important things, like an unironic love for Mandy Moore and a good grasp of key jokes in the *Arrested Development* series. He loved his family the way I love mine: like they are the world's best-kept secret.

When dinner ended, he followed me out of the restaurant, and my stomach flipped over as he placed his hand on the small of my back the way men do to their wives of thirty or forty or fifty years. The concert had already started by the time we crossed the street and walked into the venue, and I wanted immediately to be back at that table, leaning in on my elbows to hear everything this near-stranger had to say. Even today, I can still see how his face illuminated with the flash of the strobe lights that searched through the crowd in time with every song.

Most first dates only last five hours if there is sex involved, but by the time the show was over and the night was on the cusp of becoming the next day, we just weren't ready to call it quits. November in Minnesota is no place to be lingering at night, but we grabbed two cups of coffee just before the coffee shop closed and sat down on the curb anyway.

"See that?" Aaron would say three years later to our infant son as we drove through campus, pointing at the sidewalk. "That's where I fell in love with your mother. Before I smelled her armpits."

He walked me back to my car that night, where I was ready for him to throw me down on the hood. Instead, he gave me the kind of hug that men tend to give each other, the kind where a handshake sort of blends into a hug, but your clasped hands still stay between you. It is the least sexual kind of hug you can give someone, if a hug is ever really sexual, and I wondered if everything I'd felt this evening had been one-way, if I'd somehow misread the night's events to be something they weren't. Maybe this was just a friend date?

On the drive home, I intentionally missed my freeway exit just for the chance to hold my breath in a tunnel and wish along with the Smiths song I'd been playing endlessly all autumn. Let it be him.

Chapter 13

What to Do When the Person You Love Gets Brain Cancer

(or Any Cancer)

Cry.

Punch a pillow.

Punch a wall. Gently. You don't need a cancer patient *and* a person with a broken hand; that's just foolish.

Break something (not your hand; please see above). From my experience, bottles are satisfying, but I've heard fantastic things about lightbulbs as well.

Fantasize about breaking something bigger. Something that you can take a hammer to. Something you can hack apart with an ax.

Love them hard.

Love them the way they need to be loved, however that is. It is sometimes gentler than what you want to give them, because your natural inclination will be to want to squeeze them so hard their bones crack, to crawl inside them like a pod person so you never have to be apart. They may not be super into that.

Leave a note on the counter before you leave for work in the morning. Hide another in their wallet. Actually, shit, you should be doing this even if they don't have cancer. This is just good relationship advice overall. Start doing this now.

Be there.

Go away.

Treat them special and nice, like T.I., who is a modern-day poet who can guide you through the finer points of a modern romance, which is basically, uh, being super nice to someone?

Treat them like a normal person. Because cancer isn't an excuse to leave your clothes right next to the hamper when there is a perfectly good basket just waiting to be filled with dirty clothing, and the garbage still needs to be taken out. It smells. It's garbage.

There's not a right thing to do or a wrong thing to do, and sometimes there is nothing to do at all.

Okay, there is one wrong thing to do and that is Googling it. Don't Google it, okay? The Internet is good at so many things, but reassuring someone that their cancer-stricken wife/husband/son/brother/best friend is gonna be a-okay just isn't one of them.

The Internet should recognize that and just focus on its strengths (Twitter, photos of baby giraffes, online shopping) but no, it insists on housing tons and tons of "information" that will fill you with anxiety dreams where the stairs fall out from beneath you as you're climbing to the top of a tall building.

Life will unfold as it will no matter what you type into that search bar, so just give yourself a break and Google something more useful, like photos of nineties supermodels.

There aren't any right words to say or wrong words to say. Except for "God has his reasons." For the love of Pete, never say that unless you want to get kicked in the throat because no, my God is, like, "Oh, man, this sucks" while holding her hands up and shrugging. She doesn't have a reason.

You can be sad.

You *will* be sad. This is fucking sad; don't let anyone tell you otherwise.

You can be strong.

You *will* be strong. You are fucking strong; don't let your dumb brain tell you otherwise.

You will be whatever they need you to be, but more important, you will let them continue to be themselves. You will let them be sad. Or angry.

You will let them punch something (gently) or get a neck tattoo or run a marathon or just continue living their lives like average people because that is what they are.

They're not just statistics and pity cases and yellow rubber bracelets and Facebook statuses that you better share for just *one hour* to show your support, otherwise you're a cancer-loving sonofabitch.

They're people. Our people.

What do you do when the person you love gets cancer?

Your very best.

And you also cry.

Chapter 14

And Also with You

My father's dying wish was for "generations of Catholic McInernys." To be clear about the dying process, nobody asks you if you *have* a dying wish, but it's generally understood that anything you say when you are making your exit from this world to the next should be taken as explicit instructions for your children. So when the priest, wrapping up the last rites, asked my father if there was anything else he wanted to pray for, that was his answer. And while my three siblings looked at one another nervously, I felt as smug and superior as one can feel while standing at her father's deathbed, because Ralph was the only grandchild out of five who had been baptized.

We were standing in the room that had been my father's office until he went to the hospital with more chest pain than usual and ended up in the ICU. While he was lying in a hospital bed, my siblings and I had dutifully packed up the floor-to-ceiling bookshelves filled with his beautifully bound copies of everything from diet books to Faulkner. We dismantled the desk where he sat every day, writing the infomercials that would sell millions of dollars' worth of vacuum cleaners and weight loss solutions. We sanded and painted and made his dim little office a good room to die in. The paint was barely dry when the ambulance brought him home for hospice this evening and now our father is lying in a loaner hospital bed where his bookcases ought to be.

Father Gillespie, the closest thing the Archdiocese of Minneapolis–Saint Paul has to a beloved celebrity, has led us through last rites. It is the second time my father has received the sacrament, though he didn't count the first one earlier today. That priest was a free agent, some sort of hippie who floats from hospital to hospital anointing the sick. He was wearing a knit beanie when he'd parted the dark curtains of my father's room in the ICU, and I don't think my father believed a man who was dressed like he just came from an outdoor clothing sale could possibly be a priest.

At any rate, Father Gillespie is here to do it right.

Steve tries to sit up and pray with us, but the effort is too much. Father Gillespie soothes him like a child, commending his effort with a quiet *shhhhh*, a firm hand on his shoulder. On Sunday mornings I would stand next to my father in church, embarrassed at how loud he sang, how loud he prayed. I kept my voice quiet—it was hard to remember all of the words. I could never sing along with the cantor's faux-opera register, even as my father tapped his finger along the lyrics in the hymnal.

Now, Steve is moving his lips quietly beneath his breathing mask and my siblings and I are left to pick up the slack. We are awkward and self-conscious through the Hail Mary, not wanting to go too fast or too slow, not wanting to be the one to say the wrong words out loud. This is probably a residual fear from the fact that the Church recently changed the responses, a move that I believe was only done so they could see who was paying attention and

who had only been to mass once since

caught every time confidently saying "AN

while everyone around me is saying "AND W

and judging me for not keeping up with the hot

of the Vatican. Last year I'd been ambushed outside

heading to a funeral. The local news wanted to interview

about how they felt about the pope retiring. I was describe as a

"local Catholic," because they didn't really have enough space on

screen to add "goes to mass for holidays and funerals, still consid-

ers herself somewhat Catholic but has problems with patriarchy,

child sex abuse, and discrimination."

When he's led us through a series of Hail Marys so long it

becomes a meditative chant, Father Gillespie turns to me and my

siblings and asks if there are any prayers we'd like to say ourselves.

In moments like this, it's vitally important to say the right thing.

Your father will only die once, after all. Which is why I say, after

several beats of what feels to me like unbearable silence, "We're

not good at that. We don't know how to do that."

What I mean is that Catholic school did not prepare me for this

moment. What I mean is that decades of going to mass, where a

guy in front tells you what to say and when to say it, while standing

on an altar that clearly tells you who is in charge and who's zoning

out and thinking about the doughnuts in the basement, we literally

don't know what to say. We just said all the prayers we knew, like,

a hundred times. We are not cut out for freestyling. That's *your*

job, Father!

My awkward comment hangs in the air, right over our dad's

body. We are for sure, one hundred percent, letting this guy down.

And if he could talk right now, that's what he'd be telling us.

Up until just a few months ago our family dinners were char-

acterized by my father shouting, "For God's sake, we're all in the

...oom, can you keep your *goddamn voices down*?" But now that our father has collapsed back onto the bed after struggling to sit up and pray the Our Father with us, Father Gillespie gently anointing his forehead and hands with oil, we are speechless.

Father Gillespie assures me that there is not a wrong way to do it, and though my father is unable to speak, I know in his heart he is thinking, How the hell did you get through twelve years of Catholic school without knowing how to PRAY, GODDAMMIT?!

So I go for it. And I tell my dad everything I've already told him before, on Sunday afternoons as he rocked my baby to sleep, on teary phone calls from my college dorm room, on long car rides to and from college or the golf course or the grocery store. That I love him. I love him I love him I love him. That he is a good father and the best gift he has even given us is how much he loves my mother, that their happy and stable marriage has set the standard for what a loving partnership means for their four children. I am not crying. My head is clear and my voice steady. I feel like I am delivering a very important message. I am, I think, finally learning what a prayer is. It is just a thank-you.

"I love you," I tell him again and again, stroking his forehead the way he would touch my fevered head as a child. "You were such a good father to us."

"Really?" he asks me, childlike and incredulous.

"Really. I'm grateful for everything you did for us. I'm so proud to be a McInerny."

I know he hears me because his eyes are wide and he responds, his voice occluded by the respirator. I am sure that he says, "You'll always be a McInerny." Aaron hears, "But you're *not* a McInerny." One is a heartfelt, movie-worthy line and one is an ongoing joke about my being adopted/being Aaron's problem now. And you know what? Either is perfect. Because either is perfectly Steve.

Faith is a complicated thing. My father's gave him comfort and purpose. It helped that he was also in AA, which really backs you up on the whole Higher Power thing. I've learned, over the years, to cherry-pick from a lot of different areas and build my own sort of belief system. To be clear, my father was not a proponent of that. He called it Cafeteria Catholicism, and meant it as an insult. I call it Cafeteria Catholicism, and I mean it as an example of how clever I am. "Take all you want, but use all you take," my father used to say when we dished up our plates. So that's what I do. There's a lot I don't love about Catholicism, but I'll keep that out of this book to maintain important relationships with my family members. But I love the ritual of Catholicism. I love that when I step into a church in Florence, Kentucky, or Florence, Italy, it is all the same (give or take a pair of jorts). I love rows of children in identical uniforms. I love the idea of treating people well, of examining your own behavior, of trying to improve. I love the idea of a cadre of saints watching over us, just a prayer away should we lose our keys or lose our way entirely. I love that, at its best, faith gives people a specific thread to connect them through space and time, that the prayers my father said with us at bedtime were the same ones his father said at bedtime, and his father before him.

Every night at bedtime, Ralph tucks his face between my neck and shoulder and breathes me in as I draw his curtains and say, "Good night, world." We cuddle up and read books, his surprisingly elegant little toddler fingers pointing at every Spider-Man villain as he gasps, "No! Oh, no!" We say our prayers: one Our Father, one Hail Mary. Or I say the prayers and he folds his hands and says, "Prayers prayers prayers," which is a fair response to someone saying, "Let's say our prayers." We say good night to Grumpy and Papa. "Papa!" Ralphie shouts, leaning back from me with a huge smile and placing his hand over his torso. "He's in my heart!"

Chapter 15

Sorry You Dated Me

Dear [Former Boyfriend],

Remember me? Okay, don't delete this.

I hope you're doing well! That's a weird thing to write because obviously I can just stalk you online and tell you're doing pretty well, but probably no better than you were when you were my boyfriend. I'd say you're doing reasonably well, considering you once dated me.

You're probably wondering why I'm writing. No, I didn't join a pyramid scheme (yet). It's just that [length of time] has passed since our relationship ended, and I find myself reflecting on what we had. Ick, no, I don't want you back. I'm just trying to clear the air a little.

I know that I said that you were to blame for our breakup because you [smoked too much pot/didn't have a job or a savings account/had a secret girlfriend] but recently I've begun to see that I contributed to our demise through my [obsessive jealousy/ passive aggression/reading your emails].

The more I think about it, maybe you weren't a terrible boyfriend. Maybe I was actually a terrible *girlfriend,* because I [always made fun of you in front of your friends/definitely was flirting with the friend of mine you were so jealous of/tried to turn you into someone you weren't by pressuring you to stop wearing hoodies every day].

You don't need to reply to this email to confirm anything, by the way. I am already pretty sure how you feel about me since we haven't spoken since I [broke up with you while we were riding bikes/broke up with you via email/broke up with you, but still took your air conditioner].

I'll always remember our [week at Burning Man/afternoon bike rides/trip to Mexico] with [some confusion and drug-addled flashbacks/affection/fondness except for the part where you yelled at me for getting food poisoning and having explosive diarrhea].

I hope you'll find it in your heart to forgive me for [throwing out all your muscle tees while you were at work/breaking up with you over email/telling people you peed the bed when you got drunk/going on a date with your best friend] and I wish you a lifetime of happiness with [your vaporizer/whatever crust punk came after me/your wife, whatsherface].

Sincerely,

Nora

Chapter 16
Slut

I didn't know what the word meant, I just knew I didn't want to be one.

Although I wasn't in much danger of that, since I looked like the little brother from *Who's the Boss?* and my preferred look was a turtleneck under a Champion sweatshirt. But when you were eleven, you just never knew.

The slut issue had come out of nowhere. When we were ten, boyfriends were just boys who passed us notes and sometimes held our hands on the playground. But middle school was a different game, we learned. For one, we got to trade our babyish plaid jumpers for plaid skirts, which we rolled at the waist until the box pleats puffed out like tutus, revealing our Umbro shorts beneath. We started shaving our legs and mimicking the older girls, who seemed so sophisticated, like they probably had their own kids outside of school, when they weren't busy being thirteen-year-olds. We knew from whispers in the hallway that our friend's big sister had done *something* with one of the boys in her year who looked like Leonardo DiCaprio, and that now she was a slut. Just like that! It could happen to anyone. As long as you were a girl.

My friend Erica was just a geek like me, with puffy bangs and a dorky bob, and then one day she and Joey Larson French-kissed in her basement after watching *Hard Copy*. Now we were all pretty sure *she* was a slut. Other girls in our class had also kissed boys, and one had let Tyler put his hand under her uniform shirt, but over her training bra. I didn't even have a training bra. I occasionally wore a camisole under my school uniform, but I didn't even really need to. My chest was as smooth and strong as the boys' on my swim team. I'd pierced my ears just to cut down on the number of people who confused me for a boy, but it still happened, probably because I was five foot seven and wore tearaway pants as a fashion item, like I never knew when I'd be called into the big game.

But I was experiencing an awakening. I'd recently discovered some feelings in my swimsuit zone after Devon Sawa's portrayal of Casper the Friendly Ghost, where he somehow comes back to life and kisses Christina Ricci on the lips. I'd blushed in the movie theater, and then replayed the scene in my head endlessly for weeks.

My first kiss was going to be like that: just like Christina Ricci kissing a dead boy who came back to life after haunting her house. It was all very romantic, probably because I didn't have any other sexual or romantic references besides that movie and *The Little Mermaid,* which really wasn't that enticing except for the parts where Eric was washed ashore and his shirt was all wet. *Hot.*

Instead, my first kiss happened under the bridge where my friends and I had recently accidentally killed a muskrat while mindlessly throwing rocks into the creek. I spent every day after school with Justin and Andrew, boys from my neighborhood who went to my Catholic grade school and didn't acknowledge me at all during the school day, but spent every afternoon with me building forts and climbing into tree houses and doing the shit you aren't supposed to want to do anymore once you're old enough to get a boner. Other guys our age spent the afternoons trying to rent softcore porn from the video store across from school, but Justin and Andrew and I had other plans, like walking through the sewer or accidentally killing a small mammal while throwing rocks into the creek and then burying the body because we were afraid a muskrat corpse would be discovered by the police and lead to our immediate arrest.

After school, we'd go home to change out of our school uniforms, then meet up on our bikes and ride for hours around the creek and lakes around which south Minneapolis is built. The sexual tension was somewhere between nonexistent and low, but one day Justin dared Andrew to kiss me, and I felt my stomach flip around with a combination of excitement and dread. Suddenly, Andrew looked different to me. He had ridiculously long eyelashes and pink, pouty lips. Kind of like Devon Sawa, I decided.

I expected Andrew to tell Justin he was being stupid, but instead he just shrugged and said, "Okay," and then pressed his mouth to mine. I jumped back when I felt a warm slug work its way between my lips, then realized it was his tongue.

"You don't know how to kiss?" he asked, disappointed, and I felt my stomach drop. I had just been a normal girl when I woke up, but suddenly I didn't know who I was anymore, standing by the creek letting boys put their dumb tongues in my mouth? I assumed Andrew's question was rhetorical, and got on my bike, hands sweating and heart racing. It was only a matter of time before everyone knew what we'd done under that bridge, and I needed to process it for myself. I was relieved that neither of my parents' cars was in the garage when I opened the door and parked my bike. Certainly they'd notice that something was different about me when they got home, that something monumental had happened in the eight hours since they'd last seen me. I never had anything exciting to journal about, but today, I did.

Kissed Andrew today.
Am I a slut?

Chapter 17

The Game

Britney Spears had her famous meltdown in 2007, and while I now hold that version of her up as a symbol of the resilience of the human spirit, at the time it was pretty uninteresting to me because every girl I knew was losing her damn mind. Maybe we weren't shaving our heads and assaulting people with umbrellas, or maybe we *were* but nobody was there to capture it on film. Two thousand seven was the year I moved in with a bunch of girls in a two-story apartment in a South Slope, Brooklyn, row house that tilted to the right so extremely that my dresser drawers were always sliding open on their own free will. We spent Thursday through Saturday nights bouncing from bars to clubs, stopping for pizza at 4:00 A.M., and sleeping away our weekend days. I started really committing to my smoking habit, and I got a tattoo because one of my roommates, who I was scared of but wanted to like me, was getting one and I wanted her to think I was cool. "Nora," my friend Guy told me after he woke me up with a phone call at 1:00 P.M. on a Sunday, "you're like one bad night away from an *E! True Hollywood Story*." I didn't think it was fair for a guy who once pooped his pants in a Blockbuster to be throwing around judgments like that, but I told him I would let him play himself in any dramatic reenactments.

Two thousand seven was a very popular time for a really shitty book called *The Game,* which taught terrible men how to treat women terribly in order to con them into having sex. It was a really beautiful time to be a beautiful, single girl in a big city.

The premise of *The Game* was basically that if you treated a girl poorly, she'd come crawling to you. It was recommended you use a tactic called "negging," where you work a subtle insult into the conversation. Nothing too offensive, just something to knock a girl's confidence a bit. You know, like, "You have such an interesting nose," or "I've never heard of that college."

In between sifting through losers like that, I met a guy my friends and I later nicknamed the Falcon, because if you besmirch my honor my friends will try to make me laugh at your expense and because he truly did bear a resemblance to the world's fastest bird.

I was interested in him because I was interested in anyone, like that sad little bird in the old children's book walking around, asking after his mother. I was tapping any and every single New York City man on the shoulder asking, "Are you my boyfriend?" The answer was an unreturned text or, if I was lucky, a drunken make-out session in the back of the cab after which I paid the fare.

You know the part in *Gone Girl* where the crazy wife goes crazy from the pressures of being a "cool girl"? Minus faking my own death to screw over my husband, I FEEL HER. Actually, even watching that movie, I sympathized with her. That sentence alone should be a big red flag to any man who ever wants to date me, because that character is supposed to be completely insane, but I found her to be, overall, a fairly reasonable and resourceful woman.

It's *exhausting* to be a cool girl.

After weeks of flirting, which was basically me just trying to get the Falcon to laugh at my jokes while he stood around the bar with our friends, being disinterested in me, he asked me on a date. No, he asked me to hang out. Specifically, he invited me over to "watch *Arrested Development*" and "play with his kitten" (not a euphemism) and I arrived surprised to find he'd bought a bottle of Riesling and made pasta carbonara, two sure signs that a twenty-five-year-old boy is interested in you. After eating approximately three thousand calories and splitting a bottle of syrupy-sweet wine, he began to kiss me, and my lonely soul rejoiced even though he was wearing sweatpants and the size of our noses made it nearly impossible to breathe.

We never "hung out" again, but we ran into each other when our roommates, who made up the majority of my small social circle, all met up at the bar between our two apartments. "Hey," he said, tugging at my sleeve, "do you have a minute?"

"Of course!" I chirped, slamming the rest of my beer and following him out into the cold, where he told me he wasn't interested in being my boyfriend.

"I didn't even *want* a boyfriend!" I told him, shivering in my American Apparel T-shirt and cardigan combo.

I don't know where the Falcon got the idea I wanted to be Mrs. Falcon. Was it because I wanted him to chat online with me all day? Because I wanted him to be delighted by the kitten videos I emailed him at work? Was it that I sometimes texted him every day after work just to see how his day had been? Because I'd imagined our future kids' faces and then estimated the budgets for their nose jobs? Well, excuse me, buddy!

What I want to tell this girl, this sad version of myself who is walking back to a bar she hates next to a guy who looks like a very fast bird and who does not want to be her boyfriend, is that she is actually not very cool at all.

A cool girl doesn't chase boys who have secret girlfriends on the side. She doesn't follow a guy when he gets drunk, accuses her of flirting with the cabdriver, and leaps from a moving vehicle to run back to his apartment in the rain. She doesn't forgive a dude when he goes upstate to do peyote with some girls from college and forgets he's made plans with her.

A cool girl doesn't reply to a "sup" text sent at 1:00 A.M. Nothing good happens after midnight, okay? A cool girl doesn't *have* to want a boyfriend, but if she does want one, she's damn well going to get one. And it's not going to be a game.

Chapter 18

My Ex-Boyfriend's Ex-Girlfriend

I wouldn't say I was obsessed with Karen—I just knew a lot about her, considering she was a total stranger. We hadn't met personally, but I knew I hated her. I also knew her eye color, her brother's name, the last vacation she took, the names of her college roommates, and where she graduated from college.

Most of my friendships don't start with this level of research, but then again, most of my friends weren't dating my ex-boyfriend when we met. Karen was my successor, the girl I thought about while running to Beyoncé's "Ring the Alarm," even though she had met Jacob months after we broke up, when he was totally fair, single, handsome game.

Oh, like you didn't do this when you found out your ex-boyfriend was seeing someone new?

I said I didn't care who Jacob was seeing after we broke up. But of course I cared. Not because I wanted him back, but because part of me expected him to pine for me forever, probably because *The Notebook* had recently risen to the peak of its popularity, taking with it all my expectations for romantic love. But I cared who he was seeing. I cared a lot. I was jealous as hell, because she was a more natural blonde, she had bigger boobs, and she seemed to make Jacob the kind of happy boyfriend who goes apple picking, which I'd never accomplished in our eight years together.

When a mutual friend of ours mentioned that Jacob was seeing someone, I pretended to be very happy for him and not at all self-conscious about the amount of time I spent on the couch with my roommates watching *Rock of Love*. And then I locked myself in my bedroom and performed intricate Facebook forensics, clicking on friends of friends of friends to see if there were untagged photos of her that I could save to my desktop and examine to see just how much better than me she was. I was really into *Law & Order: SVU* and *The Wire* at the time, so I approached my new side project with professionalism and enthusiasm. I stopped just short of having her phone tapped and bringing in a team to enhance all her photos to look for new clues about her. But don't think I didn't consider it.

By the time I ran into Jacob at a Brooklyn bar between our apartments, I had to pretend to be surprised when he told me he was dating someone, even though I already knew that her name was Karen and that her parents were divorced and that she had gone to a much better college but had the same Hunter boots and H&M dresses I did.

After we ran into each other, Jacob emailed me to say that Karen would like to invite me out to brunch. I was stunned. What is a good detective to do when her mark invites her out for a meal? Had I been made? Had Facebook alerted her to how much time I was spending flipping through her photo albums?

I had, of course, imagined all sorts of scenarios where I would casually run into Karen and Jacob. I would, in these fantasies, be on my way to somewhere cool. A secret show by a band they hadn't heard of, or a party on a rooftop in a neighborhood they'd never go to. "How are you?" I'd ask Jacob, hugging him nonchalantly like a long-lost friend. "Oh!" I'd say, turning my warmest smile to Karen. "You must be Karen!" I would be dressed in a way that implied I looked good without trying. My blond hair would be tousled and imperfect. I wouldn't have much time to talk, of course, but I'd leave them both with the impression that I definitely had my life together, and that I was very cool. All I had to do was live out the bizarre fantasies I'd already constructed in my head. I just had to wake up, put together a decent outfit, be funny and charming, and knock both of their socks off.

Instead, I was brutally hungover from the night before. It had been a typical Friday evening spent at a neighborhood bar with my roommate Lauren, lamenting how gross it was when guys who were over thirty would try to talk to us when we were clearly just there to play skee-ball and pound beers while sharing a Parliament Light. I crossed that tender threshold between "well, I'm pretty drunk" and "holy shit, why won't my left eye open?" I'd managed to wake up early enough to put on makeup and attempt to cover the smell of stale beer and cigarette smoke with Febreze, cheap perfume, and deodorant.

Karen looked just like I thought she would look: clear-skinned and WASPy. She was definitely not hungover and had definitely showered in the past forty-eight hours. I found that as long as I sat very still, I could keep the dining room from spinning around me. For his part, Jacob spent the entire meal sweating and laughing politely while Karen and I got right down to business and started to fall in love.

In between feeling that I might vomit into my purse, I began to feel that tight knot of ugly envy inside of me loosen up and turn into the giddy butterflies you get when you're connecting with a human who you genuinely like. Karen and I both talked quickly and nervously, our life stories pouring out of our mouths in between mimosas. We both talked louder than necessary for two people who were at the same table on the same planet. We laughed at each other's jokes. We had read the same books. We liked the same music. It was like having brunch with an old friend from grammar school, picking up where you left off even though it has been years since you've seen each other. In this case, Karen and I had never met and I'd spent the better part of a fiscal quarter carefully tracking her online, but you get the point I'm trying to make.

The feminist in me cringes at the girl I was, but life is a journey, and that journey sometimes includes pit stops in Crazytown. I have yet to meet another woman who didn't take a similar detour at some point, who *doesn't* know intimate, personal details about the woman her ex-boyfriend is currently getting naked with. Or personal details about the woman her current boyfriend used to get naked with. You for sure have creeped on your ex's new lady's Instagram pics, and Britney Spears probably picks up *Us Weekly* to check on photos of Justin and Jessica and their baby. We want to know who these women are, who are so enchanting to the people we love or have loved. We want to know if they are smarter than us or more successful, or if they have a better sense of style. And the Internet, God bless it, is happy to answer those questions for us. There is a reason we clear our search history and live in fear of the day when we confuse the Facebook search area with the status area. There is a reason we have disabled the LinkedIn function that shows us who looks at our profile and lets other people see when we check on theirs: because we are checking up on one another more than we are comfortable admitting to the public or to ourselves.

Somewhere out there, there is another woman who has been naked with some of the same men you've been naked with, and you know more about her than you should. It's not your fault. Okay, some of it is. Nobody forced you to make a secret Instagram account, befriend her, and screen grab all of her pictures. That's on you.

We're conditioned to be jealous of women who come before and after us; we give them special powers and invent mythology to support how they are clearly inferior to us while harboring a fear that they are better than us in every measurable way. I pined over my boyfriends' exes more than they did, certain there was some quality they all had that would always make them bewitching and irresistible, sirens who could call my boyfriend away from me at any moment. This happened exactly zero times, by the way.

I didn't think, ever, that any of my exes' girlfriends were furiously Googling me, though I was courteous enough to leave them a healthy digital bread crumb trail of abandoned blogs and narcissistic Tumblr accounts filled with terrible writing and artistic photography to make it worth their while, just in case.

But of course they were Googling me. Admit it, ladies. You were.

Jealousy is amazing because it allows us to build fantastical worlds based purely on our own imaginations. The objects of our jealousy are almost always like an alternate-universe version of ourselves: They have something we could have, if only they didn't get to it first. We don't get jealous—really, truly, Google jealous—of people like Beyoncé or Gwyneth Paltrow. Sure, we're a little envious, but we're not lying in bed at night wondering if we'll ever measure up to them. We save that for the people we may run into at the grocery store while we're not wearing makeup. I'm not saying that it makes sense. Feelings don't make a lot of sense, which is why Taylor Swift and Katy Perry could both fall for John Mayer. Ick, right?

But like dating John Mayer, jealousy is a waste. On the other side of that boiling envy is someone who is basically just like you. Unless your exes' tastes vary wildly, you're going to find you have a lot in common with whoever got there before or after you. John Mayer only dates hot, successful women who are out of his league, and I bet any guy you've been with is the same way, so the person you're so sure you'd hate is likely just as smart and hot and successful as you are. She might, like me and Karen, probably like the same things and, more important, hate the same things as you. She might turn out to be someone who will surprise you and your husband with care packages in the mail, and help send you on a belated honeymoon when his brain tumor comes back. That probably won't happen to you, actually. But it happened to me, because that's the kind of friend Karen is. The point is, you'll find the object of your Grinch-like obsession is someone who is probably Googling you as much as you Google her, because at heart we are all just scared, insecure little humans wrapped up in Forever 21 outfits.

Jacob and Karen broke up, and he wiped us both from his life. But Karen and I? We stayed together. I have a long-distance friendship with a woman I love and cherish across many years and miles. She was there for me through my husband's chemo and radiation and death, and let me in while she went through her own double mastectomy and lung cancer diagnosis. I started out trying to learn about my enemy, and instead I found a friend. It's a goddamn buddy comedy waiting to happen. And I have my jealousy to thank for it.

Chapter 19

Who Should You Marry?

I'm so glad you asked!

First things first, marry someone funny.

No, wait. Marry someone who thinks *you're* funny, especially when you're really, really trying to be. There's nothing worse than teeing up a really great joke and having a person who *allegedly* loves you give you nothing but a polite chuckle when you were aiming for a guffaw.

Marry someone who wears your clothing size—double your wardrobe, even if there's a stack of off-limit T-shirts from his high school days that he gently explains are so precious he doesn't want you *stretching out the arms*. Laugh about that later.

Marry someone who likes the same things, sure, but, more important, hates the same things. Someone who will catch your eye in the middle of the conversation to telepathically let you know, *Yes, I heard that jackass at Starbucks try to brag to this poor barista that he is personal friends with The National and that he lives in Brooklyn like it's some far-off exotic land. We will laugh about it later until one of us pees. And that someone will be you, because you just had a baby and things are still a little out of control down there.*

Marry someone who has seen you ugly-cry.

Marry someone you like. Someone you'd want to sit next to on a cross-country Greyhound trip with no bathroom or air-conditioning, because he's the only person who could somehow make that fun and also, he's the kind of person who would have packed a snack for you.

As a rule, I don't advise people to "marry their best friend." I'm generally wary of people who tell me that their spouse is their best friend, because what happened to their actual best friend? You know, the one who prank-called boys with them in middle school and poured a beer over another girl's head in college for looking at her wrong? Did she suddenly and tragically die, or did she just get left in the dust once you found the partner of your dreams? I cannot stress this enough, folks: You are going to need to have an actual best friend because sometimes the person you marry won't agree with your DVR choices. Or, even worse, he will click on the wrong Hulu ad experience and you'll be stuck watching commercials about bone density medication when you could have been watching a commercial about lotion featuring your future best friend Jennifer Aniston. And who will you run to then? Who will you text? The animal who disregarded everything you hold dear with the click of a mouse?

Marry a person you'd marry in a church or in an art gallery. On a boat or in an abandoned factory in Russia. Someone you'd marry with the biggest blood diamond money could buy, or with a little piece of string tied around your finger. Marry someone who doesn't care about table settings or wedding favors unless *you really care about those things,* in which case, it's opposite day. Just be on the same team. Especially on your wedding day.

Marry someone brave. "For better or for worse" means promotions and babies and cancer and loss. It means having the bathtub leak into the basement because *one of you* didn't know you aren't allowed to fill a bathtub to the very top because that little metal thing on the side? That's an emergency drain. And it's broken.

Marry someone who holds his breath in every tunnel your car drives through, even when the old lady ahead of you is driving perilously slow, just so you can each make a wish that you never tell to one another *because then it might not come true.*

Marry someone who always chooses to sleep in the hospital bed with you, no matter the fact that you're both too tall for a twin-size bed even on your own.

Marry someone your parents like. Marry someone with parents who *you* like. Really, this matters, and when you're all having Thanksgiving together as a giant group and you see all of their smiling faces, you'll be glad you took my advice. Also, if your families don't get along, and you both think you were spawned from garbage people, who cares? You're making your own family, fuck 'em.

Marry someone patient. Let's face it, you're not always a walk in the park. And when you throw a fit because you can't find your keys and he says did you check your purse? and you say of course I checked my purse, do you think I'm a moron?? and then you really check your purse, and there are your keys, you want a person who will just shake his head and smile, and call you an idiot under his breath. But lovingly.

Marry a person who is perfectly imperfect, because if you've ever watched a true crime show you should know that the "perfect" spouse *always murders you in the end.*

Marry someone you admire, but more important, who admires you. If you are like me, you spent much of your twenties pursuing people who needed convincing that you were awesome. I am sorry to say that was a waste of our collagen-rich, blazing-metabolism years and that those people were never worth our time. Not when there was someone out there who would wake up every day thinking, *Fuck yeah, I married this human!*

You are worth a "fuck yeah" every day. Even (and especially) if you are still wearing your high school retainer to bed. That means you are dedicated and also frugal, two very good qualities for a person to have.

Marry a person who loves you a lot, but more important, loves you best, because quality beats quantity any day.

Chapter 20

The Most Magical Place on Earth

I went to Disney World for the first time as a twenty-nine-year-old woman. I mistakenly referred to it as Disneyland on the flight to Florida, and my husband corrected me quickly, absolutely horrified that I didn't know the difference. For those of you whose parents also didn't love you enough to take you as a kid, Disneyland is in California and Disney World is in Florida. Apparently Disney World is larger, but you still have to go to Florida to visit it, so I'm not sure that's really a selling point.

When we'd beg to go to Disney World as kids, my mom would tell us we "just aren't Florida people," as if it were a lifestyle choice and not an impossibility when you have four children. I wasn't sure exactly what that meant, but I knew it sounded better than hearing we couldn't afford it. Still, we held out hope that, like the kids in the Disney commercials, we'd wake up to a surprise trip someday.

And one day, I kind of did.

"Hello, McInerny residence, this is Nora speaking," I answered. As a seven-year-old, I was finally allowed to answer the landline as long as I stuck to the script my father had made me memorize.

"Hullo, Nora! This is Goofy!"

"Goofy?"

"Yes, Goofy! From Disney World!"

"Really?"

"Really! I'm calling to let you know that you just won a trip to Disney World!"

My legs went weak. My vision blurred. It was all happening. I was going to get the trip I'd dreamed of my entire life. The script hadn't prepared me for this, so I held the phone out to my mother.

"Mom! It's Goofy! We're going to Disney World!" I shouted, handing her the receiver and rushing to hug my little brother, Patrick, who had appeared out of nowhere at the mere mention of the Magic Kingdom. Patrick and I held each other and screamed with joy, our minds melding into a mutual fantasy of sun, fun, and photo ops with life-size versions of our favorite characters. Florida! We were going to Florida!

"You son of a bitch," we heard our mother growl into the phone, "What the hell is wrong with you? Nora, come here."

I was instantly embarrassed. My mom really had no business speaking to Goofy like this. I'm sure he very rarely handed out free vacations, and would probably be happy to give the trip to another child, one whose mother wasn't verbally abusive.

My mother handed me the phone, and I held it to my ear excitedly, ready to hash out all the details of my dream vacay with an animated dog.

"Nora, it's Mo," my uncle's voice said through the receiver, and my Florida fantasy vanished in front of me. "I was just joking! You knew that, right?"

"Yeah," I said, my voice catching in my throat, "of course!"

My Disney World fantasies dried up after being catfished by my uncle, but twenty years later, I married Aaron. A guy who had been to Disney World—or as he called it, Disney, like he was on a first-name basis with the place—*so many times he had lost count.* He was appalled that I'd never been, and after we got married, we decided to arrange a trip to the Magic Kingdom with Aaron's sister Nikki and her two beautiful children. You know, a typical honeymoon.

It took fifteen minutes to realize that my mom was right and that I really wasn't a Florida person. Humidity grosses me out, and the entire state of Florida feels like you just stepped into the bathroom after someone else showered. Only instead of knowing the steam is from your little brother or your mom, it's just the bathwater vapors of an entire state of people sticking to your skin and making your hair go limp and stringy.

Aaron had just had a brain surgery, so his doctor said that it was okay to go to Disney World, but *not* okay to ride any kind of ride that went too fast, had sudden drops, or went upside down. That sounded fantastic to me, because I don't like paying money to feel like I'm about to die, but to Aaron it was a major bummer. His idea of fun was the roller-coasters with threatening names, not riding It's a Small World four times in a row.

In spite of the fact that Aaron couldn't actually have fun and the fact that I'd chosen to wear black tights under my cutoffs to protect my skin from sun exposure, I was having a pretty okay time at Disney World. We watched our chatterbox niece turn into a wide-eyed mute as she met her favorite Disney princesses, and we watched Cinderella expertly handle the middle-aged stalker in front of us who had a photo of him and Cinderella from his last meet-and-greet printed on his crewneck sweatshirt, with the words FAIRYTALES CAN

COME TRUE. He kept telling her how they were meant to be together and she kept nodding and smiling and welcoming him to the kingdom while shooting darts from her eyes to the security guards. I got to climb into the Swiss Family Robinson tree house and see the expert merchandising power of Disney up close as every ride ended with a walk through a coordinating gift shop, where I'd find myself looking for a Nora key chain even though that has never once been an option. I could definitely see why I'd dreamed of coming here as a child, and why my parents would have opted out of this even if we could have afforded it.

After 9:00 P.M., the busiest place at Disney World was the hotel bar. We drank our iced teas and waters and watched the moms and dads around us down tequila shots and release all the stress of a long day of family fun. We'd let people think, all day, that our niece and nephew were ours. We kept them on our shoulders and sat beside them on every ride, and said thank you when people told us we were a beautiful family.

As we had left the park that day, we'd seen a woman literally foaming at the mouth while screaming at her husband to return their rental stroller as their two small children cried, clutching their souvenir mouse ears. Waiting for the bus to take us back to our 1990s hotel, we'd been the only couple without a small, weeping child in our arms. We *wanted* that.

"Aaron," I said to him in the dark of our hotel room as we fell asleep, "let's have a baby."

Chapter 21

Hot Young Widows Club

Hello, and welcome to the Hot Young Widows Club.

First, let me say that I am so fucking sorry. I wish I had something better to say, widow to widow, but I don't. I *am* so fucking sorry, and sometimes that's the only thing to say.

As you may have surmised, the cost of admission for our club is one husband. That fee is nonnegotiable and nonrefundable, a large price to pay for a club you never wanted to join in the first place. Somehow, that hasn't really affected our membership base. We do understand there has been some amount of displeasure about our fee structure, but we cannot amend it, so please direct your complaints to the Universe, God, or the friends who aren't tired of hearing you talk about your dead husband.

We do our best to make this shitty club somewhat palatable. For example, we've discovered many benefits that are available to you upon admission. These lifelong perks include making people uncomfortable in casual conversations by announcing your marital status, eliciting pity from complete strangers, and a loneliness that your friends and loved ones cannot begin to comprehend. It also includes a free pass for behaviors like crying suddenly in public places when you hear Puff Daddy and Faith Evans sing a song about losing Biggie, rage at having to fill out the "In Case of Emergency" line with a friend or parent's name, and one Widow Card, to be played only in extreme situations (e.g., "I'm sorry I was speeding, Officer. It's just . . . my husband is dead.").

Membership is for life, though you may not always be young or hot, and you may even fall in love again. We understand that.

We are unlikely to ever meet in real life, but if we do, there will be hugging.

MEET OUR FOUNDING MEMBERS

A collection of widows who promise to never ask "How are you?"

MARY

Member since: 2010
Widowed by: Brain Cancer

Mary would argue that she doesn't belong in this club, being over fifty when her husband died of brain cancer. But Mary doesn't make the rules—I do—and I say she's in, whether she likes it or not.

I skipped my first date with Aaron to attend Mary's husband's funeral. Marshall had just died of glioblastoma, a disease that was crouching somewhere inside the brain of a boy I'd yet to kiss, but would someday love and marry and lose slowly and painfully, just like Mary did her husband of so many years.

I didn't know then—neither of us did—that the very thing that stole away Mary's husband was growing within Aaron, that a year later I'd be sitting in Mary's living room drinking a glass of milk and forming an indelible bond that only comes from shared disaster or shared blood.

In the three years that Aaron was sick, Mary never told me what to feel or what to do, she just led by example: a steadfast and strong woman who kept putting one foot in front of the other, no matter how many times the path led her right off a cliff.

Mary has the uncanny ability to pop up in my inbox or on my doorstep when I most need her. She has a trial attorney's gift with words: a verbal clarity I aspire toward, while I stutter and curse my way through the tangled thoughts in my head.

It's been five years since she lost Marshall and she is starting to date. It is complicated, because dating is always complicated.

"I believe we have a sacred responsibility to live fully in the face of our losses," she tells me. "It's a bitch, though."

SAM
Member since: 2014
Widowed by: Suicide

Sam's husband hung himself in the woods near our homes in northeast Minneapolis, right before he was supposed to meet her for lunch. She was a stranger to me, but our neighborhood is a small town, and a fund-raiser for her and her toddler son had been filling my newsfeed since Sam's father and uncle found her husband down by the Mississippi.

You would not know by looking at her, sinewy and tattooed, with the hair and fashion sense that gives away her profession as a hairstylist, that just a few months ago she was destroyed, crumpled on the floor of the bedroom she'd shared with a man who'd suddenly and irrevocably decided this world was just too much for him, that his wife and child were better off alone.

"You better get up!" her father had shouted at her the day after Joseph died, as Sam lay on the floor of their bedroom. "This man left you in a world of shit, so you gotta grab a shovel!"

So she did. She sold her house a few days after his funeral and went back to work full-time. She bought a pop-up camper she named Big Bertha and takes her little dude on weekend adventures, where she is teaching him to fish while she wears plastic surgical gloves because she's severely allergic.

"My dad was *right*," Sam tells me one night, filling my wineglass while I feel sorry for myself. "You gotta get off the fucking floor and get yourself a shovel."

MARNIE
Member since: 2014
Widowed by: ???

Marnie's husband isn't dead. Not officially, at least. You can't get a death certificate when you don't have a body, but she knows she'll never find him. "He doesn't want to be found," a psychic told her, though she couldn't explain why, on a sunny summer day, Marnie's husband parked his work truck by the river and ended up in the middle of the rushing water, just above the falls in downtown Minneapolis. It must have been an accident. It had to be an accident. They were going to meet for lunch that day; he had just texted her about it, right before a stranger saw him flailing and thrashing in the middle of the mighty Mississippi.

At the search for her husband's body, Marnie locked eyes with a tall, handsome friend of a friend of a friend who had heard about the search and decided to lend a hand. Months later, when a crew showed up to rake her leaves and clean the gutters, he was there. She kissed him, on the front steps of the house she shared with her missing husband, and now she is in love with two men: one who vanished without a trace, and one who tried to find him.

Her new boyfriend goes out to dinner and drinks with Marnie and her husband's family, he picks her children up from school, he reaches out to her friends when the waves of love she feels for him are overcome by the waves of grief for her lost husband.

Their love feels hopeful because it is so inconvenient and unexpected, the way love tends to be. Maybe, I think when I see them together, I could have that again.

NORA

Member since: 2014

Widowed by: A Radioactive Spider Bite (and Brain Cancer)

I joined our club on November 25, 2014, around 2:45 P.M. I thought I was ready to say good-bye to Aaron. It had been three years of radiation and chemo and brain surgeries, and even though he was dealing with an incurable form of cancer, he insisted on being as normal a husband and father as he could possibly be, considering the circumstances.

"It's okay," I told him, rubbing his head the way I always did, "I'll be okay." Every labored breath was truly work for his body, which pressed on because that is what bodies want to do, against all odds. We are built to want to live.

I laid next to him in a hospital bed, the same kind we had become engaged in three years before, listening to his lungs and heart slowly wearing themselves out, each random and halted breath a surprise to me. And then, he didn't breathe in again. That was it. It was over. I'd seen the train coming from miles away, but it still tore me apart when it hit, the same way it tore all of these other women apart, to have the natural order of things so rudely disrupted.

This isn't much of a club, really. It's an invisible network of Internet and real-life strangers I've collected and turned into personal friends, each a reminder that I am not special, that this path has been worn by many women before me. Some of them know each other, and some of them don't. The logistics are simple: When you're in the club, you're in. And we'll find you, because we will remember how it felt to feel the earth yawn open under our feet, to have time stop and fast-forward all at once. To have people ask, "How *are* you?" when they damn well know the answer is "Well, dummy, my husband just died." We are not the first widows, nor the last; we are just walking this path together, keeping it clear for the many that have no choice but to follow in our footsteps.

On behalf of our worldwide network of members, I regretfully welcome you to the club. Please remember to check your email regularly, as we will be ordering T-shirts, and I'll need to know what size you want.

Love,

Nora McInerny Purmort

President and Founder,

Hot Young Widows Club

Chapter 22

A Letter to the Recruiter Who Emailed My Husband a Month After His Death

Dear Francine,

Thank you so much for reaching out to my husband for the senior art director position on December 8. Aaron is more than qualified for this position, and would be a great candidate for your client.

Quick question: Does this position require the candidate to be alive? I ask only because my husband has been dead for several weeks, but I don't want that small detail to overshadow his many qualifications and take him out of consideration for the job.

Please confer with your client and let me know. I can, of course, provide excellent references for my husband, though they were all from positions he held when he was alive. I'm not sure if equal opportunity laws apply to situations like this, but I can't help but think that it would be discrimination to reach out to a dead man about a job and then rescind your interest based solely on the fact that he is not currently alive. I'm not a lawyer, but it smells like a lawsuit to me.

Thanks in advance for all of your help, and have a great day!

Best,
Nora McInerny Purmort

Please note that I did not actually send this because I knew it would ruin her day.
**But I still want to send it.*

Chapter 23

Life Plans I've Made Since My Husband Died

Plan #1: Get in the car. Drive west. Perhaps stop at Culver's and get a giant root beer float. Tell Ralph we're starting over, probably in South Dakota. I've never been there, but it seems like the cure for grief is big, open skies and presidents carved into mountainsides. I can see us standing on the edge of some sort of rock formation, staring off into a sunset. We will start our new life out there. Nobody will know who we are, they will just accept this single mother into their small prairie community, and ask no questions. I'll waitress—a job I've always wanted to have but could never get the guts to do because it seems like the wrong job for someone with a poor short-term memory. We'll live in a spare apartment above the diner, which we will fill with thrift store furniture. It will always smell like hash browns.

Plan #2: Turns out that South Dakota is very cold and snowy in the winter, and I can't actually even get to Mount Rushmore right now.

Thanks, Obama. We'll put a pin in that plan until spring. What we're going to do is sell our house. Right now. Right this second. I found a tidy little brick one-and-a-half storey just a few blocks from my mother. It's a little overpriced, but I don't care. I can see just how cute it will be with an extra $100K or so to put into making the kitchen and bathroom functional, evicting all the squirrels from the attic, and replacing all the windows, the roof, and the hot water heater. We can get backyard chickens as soon as I excavate the rotting silver maple that takes up most of the backyard. It's *perfect*.

Plan #3: Okay, so apparently I don't "have the money" to buy a house and also gut it. And also, realtors recommend looking at more than one house before buying one. Also, the bank is being really annoying about the fact that I don't "have a job." *Fine*. I can see when my imaginary money isn't wanted. Ralph and I are headed west. No, not Mount Rushmore, dummies, it's too snowy. We're going to Scottsdale. Aaron's sister lives there, and after visiting for two weeks in December, I can just see us there, full-time. I can see us becoming desert people. People who go hiking and drink white wine during the day. People who like cactuses. That could be us! And why shouldn't it be? Arizona is routinely one hundred degrees warmer than it is in Minnesota, which is not even an exaggeration. What have I done in life to live somewhere there is an actual threat of losing your fingers while shoveling the two feet of snow from your walkway? Clearly, the lifestyle I *deserve* is sitting in the shade (adjacent to but not inside the sunshine), drinking white wine with my sister-in-law while our kids alternately play together and fistfight. We can punctuate that *Real Housewives* lifestyle with sunny hikes up Camelback Mountain, where we stop about two-thirds of the way up at what we call Quitter's Point, but is more aptly described as a sensible place to stop hiking when you're really high up and trying to navigate a trail that even Hobbits would have a hard time with.

Plan #4: Arizona is going to have to wait. I can't possibly expose myself to that many UV rays. I developed skin cancer during my five years as a lifeguard at the public pool. I don't know why my mother encouraged this wild Irish rose to take such a dangerous job, and I really do need to remember to blame her for this. *But you're black Irish, like your father,* she'll say when I tell her about the melanoma that originated in this small black dot, smaller than the tip of a pen, which has spread directly into my thigh, forming a tumor the size of a grapefruit that is expected to kill me in three to six months.

Plan #5: My dermatologist told that that I'm overreacting and that my skin cancer is actually "barely a freckle." You know what that means? Arizona is back on the table! I spend my nights on my iPad, browsing real estate listings and dreaming of a little cinder-block midcentury house with an updated kitchen and a citrus tree in the backyard. I even go back, a few weeks later, just to look at different neighborhoods. "I'm looking for the Brooklyn of Arizona," I tell Nikki, and I find myself asking anyone who looks remotely cool where they live. This makes for some uncomfortable situations with strangers, who apparently aren't used to being asked for their ZIP code while they're trying to enjoy a cup of coffee. It's a fact that I hate the heat, but isn't winter in Minnesota the same thing as summer in Arizona? It's extreme weather—the kind that can kill you—so you just stay indoors, where the temperature in your home and your car is engineered specifically to keep you alive in spite of your chosen climate. Big deal.

Plan #6: The Brooklyn of Arizona is my white whale. Ralph and I discuss it, and decide to put a pin in Arizona, right next to the pin we have for Mount Rushmore and for buying a new house in Minneapolis. Instead, we head to Northern California. It is clear after about two hours of temperate sunshine that this is where we are supposed to be.

"Wow," Ralph says, stepping out into another perfectly sunny day and commenting on the weather like any good middle-aged Minnesotan, "it's *perfect* today." We eat strawberries by the pound at the side of the road in Sonoma. The fruit is still warm from the sun, probably soaked in carcinogenic pesticides that will manifest themselves in a giant leg tumor, and we throw the stems on the ground and empty basket after little plastic basket of these little wonders. We sleep side by side in a tree house in far-Northern California, perched on the edge of a cliff, defying the laws of gravity and all common architectural sense. We marvel at redwood trees and we howl at the moon. This is perfect. Why doesn't everyone live in California?

Plan #7: Just found out about the drought in California and I AM FREAKING OUT. There is no water! Why do people live here? Ralph and I are going to book a flight and GTFO. This is not an appropriate place for humans to live. I'd rather freeze to death in Minnesota than die of thirst. We're going back to our house in Minneapolis, where we have enough water and no fault lines. We're gonna live there, put down our roots. And grow.

Plan #8: Except, what about New York? I *could* just move back to New York. The last time I lived there, I was in my twenties and toddlers kind of grossed me out. They were always licking the subway poles or shouting loudly at breakfast (their lunch) while I was just trying not to throw up my coffee. Kids lack any kind of empathy for hangovers. But not my kid, my kid is cool. Wouldn't it be neat to live there again, and haul an extra thirty to seventy-five pounds up and down the stairs of our walkup apartment and the subway? Wouldn't that be cute? I could be like all of those Park Slope moms I always judged when they'd dramatically wave their arms around as my friends and I smoked cigarettes in Prospect Park.

Plan #9: Okay, my friend just told me how much she pays for a nanny in Brooklyn and it is literally *five times the cost* of what day care costs here in Minneapolis. Have you ever been to Colorado? I have a few girlfriends there and I'm thinking it could be a cool place to live.

Plan #10: Just emailed a friend in Portland. Can't you totally see us living in Portland?

Plan #11: Oh my God, it's finally spring. We're heading to South Dakota.

Chapter 24

Quiet, Susan

D on't you just *hate* silence?" I asked my mom, reaching for the stereo of our Subaru after basketball practice. It was at least a fifteen-minute drive from my high school in downtown Minneapolis to our house, and my mother and I hadn't spoken since I got in the car three minutes earlier.

"No," she said, "it's nice to be alone with your own thoughts."

I took that as a sign that she was, as I'd always suspected, totally defective, and turned on 101.3 KDWB, hoping she'd let me listen to some pop music instead of the "jazz and traffic" station she insisted on listening to, like it was a good idea to combine the two most stressful things I could imagine into one radio station.

I have never been good at quiet. My parents used to read me a book called *Noisy Nora,* about a little mouse whose entire family just wants her to shut up, because people in Minnesota are not at all passive-aggressive. I didn't take the hint, and from the moment I could string a sentence together, I made sure to fill every moment with chatter.

In high school, I was the envy of at least three of my friends because I had my very own phone line and voicemail. It was a necessary safety precaution for the family, since nobody could ever get through to the house between the hours of 3:00 and 10:00 P.M., when I would take the cordless phone and spend hours curled up in my bed, talking to the friends I'd spent all day with in school, ignoring the call-waiting beeps entirely. Some mornings, I'd wake up to a dial tone, having fallen asleep talking to my boyfriend, who I also saw all day at school, but who loved to stay up talking about how cool it would be when we were grown up and married and wouldn't have to sneak down to the creek after school to find a place to kiss.

I've been busy since Aaron died. Partially out of necessity—death comes with a lot of paperwork—and partially, I don't know why. There is still a lot of noise in my life. My phone lights up every three seconds to tell me about a stranger who wants to meet for lunch, a stranger who wants to send me a loving note, or a stranger who is crucifying me in the comments section in some corner of the Internet I never wanted to be in. And then there's my own brain, which is basically an Internet Explorer window exploding with pop-ups, only instead of telling me that I've won a free vacation or offering me boner medicine, it's an exciting replay of all my character flaws and personal failures and the nagging, persistent feeling that no matter what Aaron told me, I am not going to be okay, that I am doomed to wander this earth angry and hurt and alone, like a widowed-mom version of the Incredible Hulk. For months now, my jaw has ached and my eyeballs have pulsed in my head, and I've fallen asleep and woken up in the glow of my iPhone.

Which is why I'd probably vote myself Least Likely to Go to a Silent Retreat in the Woods with No Electricity or Wi-Fi. But here

I am, sitting in my Honda Accord in the gravel parking lot, about to hide away from society for forty-eight hours.

I turned my phone off when I parked the car, but I finger it lovingly through my coat, like Bilbo Baggins with his ring, longing for its instant ability to get me out of uncomfortable situations. I'm just one button away from being transported to a world where I can lose myself in Larry Shipper theories or gluten-free bread recipes I'll never make or the baby photos of people I met once at a party five years ago.

I'm greeted at the main door of the hermitage by two short men with thick sweaters and the healthy skin of people who spend more time outside than they do in front of a computer screen. Their names immediately tumble through the detritus in my brain, then disappear altogether.

One of them leads me to a small room, where we sit in a comfortable silence for a few moments before he looks me in the eye.

"You've come here for a rest," he tells me, and I feel my face crumple into a Claire Danes cry face.

He hands me a box of tissues that appear as quickly as the rivers of mascara running down my cheeks, and I thank him.

"You know," he says softly, "even Jesus needed this."

"Tissue?"

"Silence. He went to the desert, because he needed solitude and silence to hear his own father."

I don't know what he's talking about. Sure, I went to Catholic school from kindergarten through college, but I'd somehow managed to graduate without really cracking a Bible so I'll have to take his word for it.

I nod to him and take his Kleenex, but I don't know that I'm here to hear God. I'm here for quiet, yes. I am here for a rest, yes. And this does happen to be a hermitage run by a bunch of Christians.

But that doesn't mean I'm here to talk to God, buddy. I'm just here to sleep in a twin bed in a cabin with no electricity and no Netflix.

In general, religion falls into a category of Things Not to Talk About that also includes workout habits, dietary issues, and dreams, so I really don't want to talk God with this guy just because I decided to come to a religious retreat center. I'd actually like to talk with nobody, because I thought that was kind of the point of the weekend. But if God does show up, I suppose I can't exactly stop him.

This man, and I still can't find his name anywhere in my head, so let's just call him Buddy, grabs my overpacked bag and throws it in the back of his truck. It's a very short drive to my cabin, just past the sign that requests you observe silence. It's a sweet, nondescript little place. Just one room, with a screened-in porch attached. Inside, it's like any dorm room from college, minus the running water, electricity, or the stash of Mike's Hard Lemonade under the bed (I checked). One rocking chair faces a big picture window, which opens onto the prairie.

I have never looked out a window as clean as this one, so spotless it is as if the glass does not exist.

Buddy hands me a small basket with a block of cheese, two apples, and an orange. There is no fridge, I realize, because those tend to run on electricity, so I open the side door and set the basket on the screened-in porch. Sometimes, Minnesota is its own refrigerator. I feel like that could be our new state motto. Someone from the government—call me. I make a mental note to tweet that when I leave, and Buddy tells me that dinner, if I care to join, is at five o'clock, four hours from now.

"You know," he tells me as he puts his hand on the doorknob, "we all carry something with us. Something too big for ourselves. Something that keeps us from hearing God." He gestures to a small altar adjacent to the window. "It seems silly, but write it down. Put it there."

It does seem silly, but that's what I do when he leaves, because I realize quickly that there is nothing else to do and I have made a mistake dedicating forty-eight hours of my life to this when I could be watching old episodes of *Real Housewives* or getting lost in YouTube looking for toy commercials from the nineties. The hermitage website had instructed me not to bring any books or devices, and I love rules, so I had obeyed them. Which left me alone in a ten-by-ten cabin with no electricity and nothing but a notebook and a Bible and a rocking chair, counting down the minutes until I could rejoin normal society and Twitter.

By the time I've written down all my feelings and laid them on top of a Bible, there is literally nothing else to do in this cabin, so to fill some time until dinner, I try to pray, and find there are so many other words clunking around in my head that I've created a remix mash-up of the best parts of the Our Father and the Hail Mary.

I eat both of my apples and half a block of cheese and try not to look at the little clock next to my bed.

It has been seventeen minutes since Buddy left me in this cabin, which means I have forty-seven hours and forty-three minutes to go.

I decide this is a good weekend to learn how to do a handstand, and push all the furniture to one edge of the cabin so my giant body has enough room to invert itself. My arms are tired, which means I must have been doing this for hours.

It has been five minutes.

I stopped for a giant coffee on my way up here, and now I have to use the bathroom. But . . . there isn't a bathroom, which should have been obvious when they said there was no running water, but wasn't, because I am an idiot. I just assumed that they were exaggerating, and there wouldn't be showers available. I didn't anticipate each trip to the bathroom including a hat, gloves, and parka, but at least the process takes up about five minutes if I walk as slowly as possible.

I'm not a napper, but at this point I have to do something to burn some time, so I lay in my little twin bed, close my eyes, and hope for the best. When I wake up, I know I've been asleep for days.

It's been twenty-three minutes.

If you're bored just reading this, *good,* because that is how I felt and I must be a really good writer to make you feel my feelings, right? After sitting alone in my cabin debating whether I should just run to my car, spend the next two nights alone in a hotel room watching Bravo and eating fast food and telling people the retreat was "transformative," I leave for dinner at 4:45. It only takes five minutes to walk to the lodge, so I am awkwardly early, just the way I like it.

There is a fire roaring in the fireplace, and for a moment I don't even notice my dinner companion. I'm thrilled that Kristen Wiig has chosen to go on a spiritual retreat in Minnesota the same weekend I am, until I realize that this woman is not Kristen Wiig, she is just the personification of her Target Lady character.

"Hi," she says, "I'm Susan, and I'm a CHRISTIAN." I'm familiar with the term, but Susan says the word in all caps, like I may not have heard it before. She wants to know if I am a CHRISTIAN and she nods in approval when I tell her that I was raised Catholic. She offers me the use of some of her contraband books while I'm up here. She knows you're not *supposed* to bring any books, but because she only reads CHRISTIAN nonfiction, a genre I didn't know about, she thinks it is probably okay to bend the rules a bit. Susan spends our time together until dinner providing me with many opinions on a variety of CHRISTIAN topics, and by the time we are welcomed to sit down at the table, my face and neck hurt from nodding and smiling, and I am longing for my stupid little cabin and its maddening silence.

Dinner is hosted by two hermitage employees, sweet, simple people who are probably not tempted to roll their eyes while Susan continues her monologue about her CHRISTIAN dog-training business. When I turn down the rolls because I can't eat gluten, the woman who cooks dinner lights up.

"You know," she tells me, pointing her roll at me for emphasis, "we had another guest here with a *severe* gluten allergy. But she loved the smell of this bread—who wouldn't!—and she *prayed* and *prayed* to God to just relieve her allergy . . . just while she was staying here."

She pauses for dramatic effect and I cannot tell if this is a joke or a serious story, so there is not even an emoji I can use to reflect my facial expression at this point.

"And you know what? *He listened*. Whenever she visits . . . her allergy goes away, and she can eat bread and muffins with no problems. *None*."

I nod emphatically, because it is more polite than explaining to somebody with a good heart and good intentions that the God who was apparently up here granting muffin-related miracles had kind of dropped the ball on giving my husband a waiver for his brain cancer, and we had for sure asked for that.

I eat my iceberg lettuce and baked chicken quickly and quietly because Susan shows no signs of slowing down, and she's just getting started on the evils of the Internet when I have to excuse myself to return to the personal hell that is my cabin.

It is dark when I leave for my cabin, and I realize as soon as I step onto the wooded path that I forgot to memorize my way back before the sun set.

The weak beam of my flashlight shows me only the few feet in front of me, just snow, snow, and more snow, with footprints from people and animals that led in infinite directions. I start on the path, but soon I'm not sure that I'm still on it, and the sight of my cabin is a complete surprise when it pops up in front of me. I'm overcome with relief at the sight of these four stupid walls, even if there is no electricity or Wi-Fi inside.

Inside my little cabin, I am almost happy. I light the gas lamp and brush my teeth with a pitcher of water and a basin, like Laura Ingalls Wilder but with a Sonicare. From my little rocking chair, I can see headlights making their way down a distant road, then disappearing back into the darkness. That noisy world—and Susan—are closer than they appear, and in forty hours or so I will return to my normal life and all the tweets and emails that are piling up during my hiatus. I realize after a few moments of rocking in my chair that I haven't heard a thing, that my brain is as quiet as this cabin. And I don't hate the silence.

Chapter 25
Madge

My mom is my mom.

And by that I mean that like most women, I love and adore her and also she drives me insane and there is a very real risk of my elder-abusing her in a few years, given the right circumstances. The wrong circumstances? Either way, watch out, Madge!

Some women are going to read this and say, "Not me! My mother is my *best friend*!" To which I say, keep telling yourself that. Because I'm not afraid to admit that sometimes my mother breathes and I can hear the air moving through her nose and suddenly all the love I've ever felt for her just dissolves into a puff of smoke. And sometimes I see her and I love her so much my heart could explode. But then she asks me if I'm planning to get a haircut soon and I need to go into the other room and take five. But *then* she plays with the ends of my hair while I watch TV, and I feel like I am seven again and she is the most perfect human I've ever met.

The love we get from our parents is not completely unconditional.

It's impossible for it to be, because before you even *have* a child, you have fantasies about who he or she will be. In the early stages of love, you look at your partner and say things like, "Oh, gosh, our kids are going to be so cute. And I bet they'll be good at math and love golf, like me. And they'll have a funny upper lip, just like you." So a child is born into a nice warm pool of expectations, and while your parents will love you no matter what, the fine print reads that they will love you *more* if you turn into the person they imagined you to be.

I knew as a child that my mom had some idea of who I should be and how I should get there. Madge was always very interested in showing me how to do things. That is different than teaching someone how to do things, which is difficult with children because they aren't good at anything, and it is easy to lose your patience and just do it for them. Which is basically how I remember my mother: standing behind me, holding my hand and guiding a paintbrush across the paper; holding both of my hands and knitting, then purling. Sometimes it was frustrating, but sometimes it was kind of awesome, like when I was ten and she took my school report on Minnesota, ripped it out of the plastic cover I'd bought at Walgreens, and bound it with leather and birch bark. I didn't just get an A, I got sent to the state fair, where my mother won a blue ribbon. Sometimes it was benevolent and lifesaving, like when I was fifteen and finally got my period, a year after I lied about getting it to fit in. I had just read the warning brochure that comes with every box of tampons and was convinced I was going to die of toxic shock syndrome, and I couldn't get my tampon out. Nothing had ever been up there before, so it was really wedged in, and also, you do have to apply some pressure when you're pulling on a string attached to a cotton plug that has soaked up your uterine lining. I was crying in the bathroom, imagining how embarrassed

I would be at my own funeral with everyone knowing that I died of tampon disease. When Madge knocked on the door to tell me to quiet down, I told her what was happening, and prepared to die of embarrassment. But Madge opened the door, reached over, pulled it out for me, and *never mentioned it again*. Like a boss.

My dad was strict and intimidating, but he wasn't the boss of our family. Madge was our boss. She had veto power over all of our father's decisions, which was good because his default answer for every question was just no. Madge had a full-time job but also managed our father's finances as he grew his freelance career. I think just knowing in her heart that she had the power to uproot and run away with all the money really got her through the trying times of raising four children with a man who would write her love poems but also ask her every night when she returned from work, "Where is my dinner?" As if it had gone missing, and only a woman could find it for him. When shit went down and you were caught trying to sneak into the house after midnight buzzed on a few Mike's Hard Lemonades, it might be our dad who threatened to knock you into the middle of next week, but it was our mother who would break you down with a cold, icy silence that told you just how disappointed she was in your existence. She could be harsh, but fair.

I was afraid to learn how to drive, but she encouraged me from the front seat of her brand-new SUV as I lurched around our neighborhood, slamming on the brakes every few seconds and wondering why people chose to drive when walking and biking were so much easier. "Go ahead and pull it into the garage!" she said when I pulled into our driveway, dripping sweat. Our house had been built in 1932, so the tuck-under garage wasn't exactly spacious, but I squeaked us in without scraping the sides. And then I forgot which pedal was the brake, and made a game-time decision just to

142 - It's Okay to Laugh

pick one, which ended with our new car smashed into the cinderblock foundation of our house. My dad popped up out of nowhere, screaming about how I shouldn't have smashed the car into our house, but my mom calmly locked our car doors and put the car in "park" for me. "Don't worry, you'll get the hang of it," she said, and traded her fancy SUV for a very safe, very sturdy Subaru.

No matter how much you love and admire your mother, you don't always want the wisdom she is so eager to share, especially when you're a woman. It goes back to that whole wanting to kill her just for breathing wrong thing, which most men I know don't feel about their moms. Woman to woman, we want to be able to assert who we are apart from the woman who raised us and the choices she made. We don't want her rearranging our cabinets or giving us diet tips or telling us that she doesn't care for our boyfriend. We don't want her opinion until we want her opinion, and at that point we just want her to agree with us.

Our relationship has had several hiccups, where I have been convinced that my mother no longer loves me at all. I'm prepared to take responsibility for the few months she ignored me in college after I thought it would be funny to create a very elaborate hoax where my boyfriend and I convinced my parents we were dropping out at age twenty to get married. We'd started the prank a few weeks before, for maximum effect, and the "punch line" was delivered through a letter that arrived on April 1, and told them they were dummies for believing us. Unfortunately, my parents had already begun damage control phone calls to our extended family to tell them about the upcoming nuptials. I can see now that I should have instead faked a pregnancy.

But at twenty-six, when she closed me out of her life because my boyfriend just wasn't good enough for me, *in her opinion*? Not super-chill. And looking back, no, he wasn't marriage material.

But neither was I. And every one of those hearts I stepped on got me right to Aaron, so wasn't it worth it? I returned to her, contrite, and with evidence that I had shed the offending boyfriend, and she opened up the little Nora-shaped space in her heart and let me back in for weekly yoga sessions and Sunday brunch.

This is a phase I thought I would grow out of, but nope, I'm thirty-two and I just want my mother's approval. It is a bit easier to come by these days. Not because I am so much older and more mature because I do still wear my retainer to bed, but because my mother and I share a category that most of her friends won't even occupy for many years. We're both widows.

My father died just six weeks before my own husband did, their cancers eating them alive and leaving just gray, hollow shells behind. We lost the same two people in very different ways. I lost the future I expected with Aaron, and she lost the man she'd spent most of her past with. I lost my father and my husband, and she lost her husband and her son-in-law. We are carrying our grief differently, but we show up for each other in ways that the rest of the family just can't. I know, when I see her pause at the bookcase or stare into her morning cup of coffee, that she is somewhere else, off exploring the alternate universe of what could or should have been. When she returns from her time travels, her eyes are wet and she gives me three squeezes: *I. Love. You.* When I tell her I am moving to Arizona— no, California—or that I am going to get Ralph a dog—no, some chickens—she just smiles and says, "That sounds great." When I tell her I had a postmortem chitchat with Aaron after he died, and that he told me I need to move out of our house, she clears out two rooms for me and my son, and we become roommates once again. When I tell her I got a little drunk and made out with a guy in a van, she laughs, even though when I told her the same story at twenty-four, she shook her head and told me to grow up.

This is progress, right?

For once she is not here to share her advice with me, or to hold my hands and guide me through it until I've reached competency. I don't have to live up to her expectations, because she doesn't have any, because she has only been a widow six weeks longer than I have, and six weeks is not enough time to get any sort of proficiency in a new life. Widowhood, living without the person that you have chosen to share your life with, is not something either of us knows how to do. We can only try to learn from each other, show each other how to survive, and love each other somewhat unconditionally, some of the time.

Chapter 26

It's a Secret, So Hush

I know what I'm seeing before she tells me.

I knew when the midwife excused herself from the examination room, claiming not to be an ultrasound expert. I knew when the ultrasound tech looked at the screen and recommended we move to her room, where the machinery is more advanced. I knew when I saw her face, and the tiny white figure hanging motionless on the monitor.

I knew the night before, even before Googling, that no blood is good blood when you're pregnant. I called the twenty-four-hour nurse line, curled up in bed, with Aaron beside me playing with the ends of my hair and tracing an infinity symbol between by shoulder blades. "It's not *blood*," I tell her, "it's just, blood-ish. Like, it's more gray than pink." Never in my life have I paid such attention to anything that's come out of my vagina, including the very alive child who is sleeping in the room next to ours.

"If you're not in pain," she assures me, "you're probably not having a miscarriage."

I close my eyes and try to listen to my body, but I can't hear a thing above the noise in my brain.

It's gone.

You wanted too much.

Ralph will never have a sibling.

You should have been happy with what you had.

Aaron doesn't need this right now.

It's gone. It's your fault. You made a mistake. You wanted too much.

My father once described the ultrasound photos I provided of Ralph as "an invasion of a baby's privacy" and asked not to see any more of them. I don't know if this is a standard practice for Libertarians, or just a typical contrarian response from my dad, but I respect it. Babies dance along with the ultrasound machine, like a little alien trying to avoid detection, a little white whale darting around your uterus hiding from Captain Ahab, a little marionette with invisible strings.

But not this baby.

"I'm sorry," the ultrasound tech said slowly and quietly, "your baby just isn't alive."

Alive is a very important aspect of being a baby, and I hoped she had a really good "but" to follow that sentence: "but it will be! Just let me see here . . ."

There was no "but."

I roll my head away from the monitor, toward the drop-ceiling tiles and the window that looks out onto a suitably gray afternoon. Outside it is raining, a brisk October rain that has brought out the sweet smell of decaying leaves and the impending chill of winter. Aaron had an MRI at seven this morning, an ungodly hour that leaves him fading and exhausted in the passenger seat outside of the clinic.

"You can stay in the car," I tell him, "it'll just be a few minutes."

"No, I should come in," he says, trying to unbuckle his seatbelt while his left arm hangs lifeless in its sling.

"No, no. Really. It'll be fine. You should listen to your show."

He kisses me and taps my nose with his pointer finger.

"Boop. I love you, Norn."

There are many women in and out of that room. Perfect strangers, these medical professionals, hugging me closely, their tears finally turning on my own emotions until my cheeks are in their full Irish mode: red and splotchy, hot to the touch.

Can you come up here, darling? I text him, and fifteen minutes later, there's a knock at the door.

I don't know when it happened, when the butterfly heart I'd seen at eight weeks turned to the ghost inside of me. What was I doing not to notice something so monumental? Driving my car, shopping for groceries, eating a bowl of cereal in bed—none of these seem like the things that should keep a mother from noticing her baby no longer is.

He needs help getting the door open. His left arm has stopped working entirely, and his left leg recently followed suit, dragging a bit as he walks. I've begun tying his shoes in the morning, fastening his belt, which has moved in a notch. Even behind his dark, thick-rimmed glasses his eyes are puffy and tired, his giant head balanced precariously on a rail-thin body.

"I'm sorry," I tell him, because that's what I am. For all of this.

There's a secret passageway for women like me: They don't lead you past examination rooms filled with round women waiting to be told how well their babies are growing. They lead you back through a maze of beige hallways, to an office where you and your husband can sit side by side in two armless chairs like insolent teens waiting for the principal.

My midwife is crying when she opens the door. A year and a half ago, she'd delivered our Ralph, and I'd learned after chatting with her between contractions that she lived next door to one of my best friends when I was growing up. Kate and I spent our Saturday afternoons playing Desert Island, a game where two aristocrats (me and Kate) washed ashore on a desert island (her unmistakably deciduous backyard in southwest Minneapolis) with their servant (Kate's little sister, in charge of grabbing us snacks from the kitchen when we were tired of foraging, aka poking around in my future midwife's backyard and mashing leaves from her plants into "soup" we pretended to cook in five-gallon ice cream pails).

My midwife has the sweet face of a good Minnesota woman: naturally flushed cheeks and clear, bright eyes, an unfussy natural beauty that comes with over thirty years of ushering life into this universe, and sometimes watching that life flicker out before it can arrive.

"There's nothing you could have done," she tells me, and I want to believe her, but I know, somewhere inside of me, that she is wrong. Everything is *someone's* fault, and who else could be to blame but the person whose biological responsibility is the creation of life? Even my father can't blame Obama for this one.

I just want to know what to do, and she lays out my options:

1. Go home and let your body miscarry naturally. As much as I'd love to spend the next two to five days waiting for my dead baby to bleed its way out of my body, I politely decline.

2. Take a pill, go home, and let my body miscarry. Again, not for me.

3. Get what is basically an abortion, but for dead babies. They can do it tomorrow. I tell her I will be there at 8:00 A.M.

There's only one way out of this place, though, and that means through the waiting room. I put on lipstick and run my fingers through my hair before we open the door, buttoning my coat in case any of these women can somehow see by looking at me that I've failed at my genetic duty. Everyone stares at us, but only because Aaron has the gait of a zombie, and holds my shoulder to steady himself while we navigate through a maze of poorly upholstered 1980s waiting room chairs. They are the same ones your doctor has, and every doctor in America. I imagine that every medical license also comes with a collection of bland upholstered chairs.

"Fuck," I say as we walk down the cold, gray parking ramp, "I have to call my mom."

I fasten my seatbelt and turn the key in the ignition.

Nothing.

I vaguely remember the gas light coming on when we'd pulled into the parking ramp.

"Oh, shit." Aaron says, "I turned the car on while I was waiting for you because I was cold and we ran out of gas. I totally forgot."

When I stop laughing and wipe the tears from my eyes, I call AAA. They're thrilled to hear from me, and to let me know that our membership expired two weeks ago.

I'm out of options, because calling any of our friends means telling them not just that we've run out of gas in a hospital parking ramp, but that I just miscarried a baby they knew nothing about. So, five minutes and one credit card charge later, we're once again card-carrying AAA members and a tow truck is on its way with a gallon of gas.

I'M FILLED WITH SECRET SORROWS. Across the city, my father is dying in the intensive care unit of another hospital. He was diag-nosed with cancer of the everything in May, when an oncologist told him he'd have six months to live if he skipped out on chemo. We're nearing the five-month mark, and despite chemo, he's withering away in a hospital bed in a first-ring suburb. Nobody knows he's sick, really. He's a marine at heart, still, stoic and strong and not about to be a bother to anybody. "I don't want to make a big deal of this," he told my siblings and me, all lined up on the floor of my parents' living room, cross-legged, confused as kindergartners being told that Santa doesn't exist. "I don't want anyone talking about this."

This being a cancer that has carved out its invisible infrastructure within his strong, healthy body, colonizing his esophagus, his lymphatic system, his lungs.

Aaron's seizures, once a crazy, once-in-a-blue-moon kind of thing, are a regular occurrence now. "Nora!" he'll shout. "I'm going down!" And I'll rush to his side and tackle him onto our bed, a sofa, or any soft surface I can find.

After a seizure, his nose conjures fragrances from out of nowhere, a side effect of all the chemicals in his brain releasing willy-nilly. "Who's frying onions?" he asks me disgustedly as he regains control of himself after the hostage takeover his brain just pulled on his jerking, helpless body, as if while I was scratching his back and calling 911, I'd also had time to put on a pan of fragrant white onions, just for the occasion.

THE DAY OF OUR HORROR show at the midwife's office, Aaron's oncologist had conservatively told us that Aaron's brain wasn't getting any better, and was maybe getting worse. The picture of his brain, a blurry black-and-white image on a PC screen, had more white than it should, evidence that despite the air strike of chemo and radiation, we were fighting a war on terrorism that could not be won. These are facts that Aaron wants to keep to ourselves, so I had tucked them away next to the pain of my father's secret cancer and the tentative joy of our secret second baby.

Culturally, we train ourselves not to speak of pregnancies before the twelve-week mark, but after an ultrasound at eight weeks, we'd slowly spilled the beans to our family. I ordered a T-shirt for Ralph that read BIG BROTHER in bold, bright letters, and some maternity leggings for myself.

We've all bought into the power of the jinx, that the only way to usher a baby safely into this world is to make sure you just don't get your hopes up too high. I jinxed it with that order from Old Navy, so this is my fault.

I've spent weeks being sad for my father and sad for Aaron, each of them volleying me back and forth across the city in a selfless game of Ping-Pong, assuring me as they fade before my eyes that they are fine and my time is best spent with the other.

But now, I am sad for this baby.

It's a new kind of sadness to feel. It's not for myself, and it's not a typical brand of mourning, either. It's cold comfort to know how many women have been here before. How many women I know. How many women around the world heard the same news on this same day, felt the same perceptible loss of something that almost was. Almost is always the hardest, isn't it?

They and I have all felt the throat full of jagged glass, the boiling of tears behind our eyelids, the sudden presence of a mysterious, age-old sorrow that stitches us together into the invisible patchwork quilt of love and loss. I hope like me that they all have a child at home to cling to, though I know many of them do not, and for those women I cry just a little bit more and whisper the only prayer that makes sense: "I'm sorry. I'm sorry. I'm sorry."

"For what?" Aaron asks, and I'm unaware I was even speaking aloud.

"For everything," I tell him, and open the car door to flag down the tow truck.

SOMETHING LIKE 20 PERCENT OF pregnancies end in miscarriages, and carrying the joy of a secret baby within you doesn't prepare you for the sorrow of a secret loss. If you lose a baby, and nobody knew about it in the first place, does it make a sound? You're damn right it does. It's a deafening loss, in a pitch only your ears can hear. When you open your mouth and tell people about that hole that was punched through the center of your heart, you'll be surprised at who comes to fill it, at how many women raise their hands and say, "Me, too."

The day I found out about my second pregnancy, my friend lost her second pregnancy. It was just a little bit of blood, and then a lot. It was hours of pain, another labor for a baby just a few weeks along. Amid the blood and internal wreckage, she'd found her child, the size and shape of a small shrimp, and buried it outside in her garden.

I carried with this second child the sorrow of my friend's loss, and a bitter sense of irony as my own body swelled with life while Aaron's waned beside me. We lay together in a rickety bed in an A-frame cabin in northern Minnesota, Aaron nauseous from chemo, me from morning sickness. It was August, but the forest was so damp and cold it felt more like March, and we slept like the dead under layers of wool blankets, waking only when Ralph kissed both our faces and said, "Morning, guys."

If you're reading this, you're one of the 80 percent of zygotes who made it all the way into this world. Do you know what that means? It means you did it! You are supposed to be here. You're incredible. You're a fucking miracle. Try every day to remember that, when you are confronted with jerks or people who don't use their turn signals. We all got here. We're alive on this planet, this mote of dust suspended in a sunbeam, against all odds. And also, please use your turn signal.

Just before all of this, I was reading Anne Lamott's *Traveling Mercies,* unknowingly preparing myself for weeks of impending heartbreak. The night before I would lose this baby, this paragraph would leap from the page and embed itself in my brain.

> *". . . when a lot of things start going wrong all at once, it is to protect something big and lovely that is trying to get itself born—and that this something needs for you to be distracted so that it can be born as perfectly as possible."*

Anne, you better be right.

Tomorrow, my sister will pick me up and a doctor will remove this baby from my uterus. It will be as if it never happened. In a week, my father will die in a makeshift bedroom we've created in his former study. In a month and a half, I'll dress my husband's dead body in his favorite J.Crew clothes and send him out the door with two handsome young undertakers.

Someday, I will see where this led me, and it will make a little more sense, but it will always, always be sad, and I will never forget that wraith of a figure, still as stone, a little shadow within me.

I am done trying to reason with it. For now, at least. There is no reason. There is nothing to understand. There is no could-have or should-have because there is only what is. What happened is the only thing that could have happened: this little human was not meant for this world, but gave it a try anyway. My father got sixty-four years. Aaron got thirty-five. And I don't have to like it, but I can't change it, either.

I talk about it because none of it needs to be a secret, and because I don't want to forget any of it, even the parts that were hard to watch. I'm proud to have kept my eyes open when it would have been easier to look away. I'll carry forever the images of our lifeless child suspended in the darkness of my own womb, my mother leaning over to kiss good-bye her husband of forty years, my husband politely apologizing for "ruining dinner" while his body jerks under the power of a seizure. The last time Aaron told me he loved me, he was lying in a hospital bed in what used to be our office, gazing adoringly at me in my retainer and L.L.Bean pajamas. Those three words were the last he ever spoke to me.

These are the diamonds I picked from the darkness, that shine with meaning only for me.

Chapter 27

Immaculate Conception

I took my first pregnancy test when I was sixteen, in the bathroom of a Walgreens six miles away from my parents' house. There was a Walgreens just half a mile away, but buying a pregnancy test literally in the shadow of my Catholic grade school was simply too risky. I was guaranteed to be seen by someone's mom or brother, even if I tried to conceal the telltale box with a *Seventeen* magazine and some two-for-one M&M's.

So instead, I drove my mother's lime green VW Beetle to the nearest suburb, a hot pink, plastic gerbera daisy bobbing its head in the dashboard bud vase.

This was 1999, before every child was born with an iPhone in its hand, so I had nothing to do but wait with my own thoughts for every agonizing minute until the test decided my fate.

How would I tell my parents? I wondered. How would everyone react? How rare, exactly, was it for a virgin to get pregnant besides Jesus' mom?

To my shock and delight, my test was negative. Probably

(although I'm not going to pretend to be some kind of medical professional, so please do not consider this medical advice) because I *was* a virgin. Most virgins aren't extremely concerned about unplanned pregnancies, but our friend's mother, who was a registered nurse, had recently given us all a real cold shower of a talk. She swore up and down that she'd just delivered *twin* babies to a fifteen-year-old mother in St. Paul who was a virgin. A virgin! Her patient had thought she was safe as long as she didn't have penis-vagina sex but she learned the hard way that nope, that was not the case, and she sure wished she had just stopped at kissing.

Typing this story out now I realize that his mom was just trying to keep us innocent and prevent her son from becoming a teenage father, but instead she drove me to an obsessive belief that I was always pregnant.

After scrutinizing the results for approximately ten minutes to make sure I hadn't misread them, I was satisfied with the veracity of the test. I wrapped the little plastic wand in about six pounds of toilet paper and buried it in the garbage can, hoping it couldn't be traced back to me in any way should a curious custodian happen to see the vague outline of a pregnancy test through the garbage bag and, surmising it had come from a wayward youth, decide to call the cops, who would immediately run some DNA testing on it and then find my parents and tell them their daughter was a Grade-A SLUT. You just can't be too careful.

My mother probably deserves some of the blame for this hysteria, if only because I like to blame her for most things in my life. She'd told me and my first boyfriend, who she once caught kissing me on the couch after school, that if we had sex, we would *without a doubt* get pregnant.

"I've had four kids," she told him as he contemplated jumping out our dining room window mid-lecture, "and both of Nora's grandmothers had nine. *Nine.* She comes from a long line of fertile women."

I wasn't going to take any chances, so I started birth control before I even started having sex—*just in case*—and still anxiously awaited the arrival of my period every single month.

Poor teenage Nora would be relieved/sad/confused to know that I didn't eventually get pregnant from kissing. I didn't even get pregnant from having sex.

I got pregnant from science.

After Aaron's diagnosis, right before he started treatment, I asked Aaron's oncology nurse about having babies. They'd already cautioned us against unprotected sex, or as they sensually described it, "the exchange of bodily fluids," and I could hear her shift uncomfortably on the other end of the phone before telling me how unpredictable and challenging this disease would be for him. But that's not what I called to hear, so I asked again and she recommended he take a visit to a nearby "cryogenics lab" before he began radiation and chemotherapy.

While it sounds extremely fancy, a cryogenics lab is just a fancy term for *sperm bank,* which is just a fancy term for a battered, vaguely medical office in a suburban strip mall. This particular one was wedged between a closed bookstore and an insurance office. The lab was a perfect example of just how misleading a website can be: there are no perfectly polished and smiling nurses in lab coats, no handsome and eligible young Ivy Leaguers in the waiting room waiting to donate some sperm to a couple in need. Just a red-eyed guy with a breakfast Mountain Dew who takes your insurance information, and a few weathered and meth-faced guys in beat-up Caprices in the parking lot who I would pay to keep their sperm away from my vagina.

Aaron had a half dozen doctor's appointments that week, a

hundred ways for them to poke and prick and examine him before they treated him, but he still woke up at seven to jerk off in a strip mall closet so we could have a family someday. That's love.

I once saw the nurse who got me pregnant while I was standing in line at the airport. It took me a while to place her, which I hated, because I'd like to think I could quickly name all the people who have ever seen my vagina, let alone the number of people who have inserted a small syringe of sperm into it. That syringe of sperm had ended up turning into a positive pregnancy test that had turned out to be Ralph, who was now sitting like a prince in an expensive running stroller, with his own ticket to Arizona, earning miles on his own frequent flier account.

"All right," I had said to her on that April morning two and a half years ago, spreading my legs and closing my eyes, "go ahead and get me pregnant." I'd kissed Aaron good-bye that morning and let him sleep off the chemo while I headed off to be inseminated before starting my workday.

She nailed it. I was totally pregnant, and it was all thanks to her, and to the pregnancy pact I made with my two childhood friends. Never doubt the power of a pinkie swear made at a wedding reception when you're all kind of buzzed. I had always planned to send my nurse a thank-you card for impregnating me, in which I said all the right things and thanked her for her hand in creating the small human whose dragon breath wakes me up every morning with a terrible-smelling but achingly sincere "I love you, Mama," breathed directly into my face and followed with a wet, open-mouth kiss. But it turns out that card doesn't exist, and no matter how I tried to catch her eye as we wound through an endless TSA line, I couldn't make it happen. I also couldn't remember her first name, so I didn't know what to yell, and "Hey! Hey! You got me pregnant!" seemed like it might be a little too aggressive for an airport. So instead I will consider this paragraph as my thank-you card, and hope that she reads it in the break room while she rests between impregnating other women and making their dreams come true.

I also hope that my friend's mom is reading this, because she was right: you *can* get pregnant without having sex, it's just going to cost you a little more than dry-humping your boyfriend in the front seat of his parents' Lincoln, and it will involve a series of strangers becoming very intimate with your swimsuit zone. The medical community calls it IUI, but I call it immaculate conception. Because it's a fucking miracle.

Chapter 28

Helpful Advice for New Mothers

A COLLECTION OF UNSOLICITED TIPS AND TRICKS FROM TOTAL STRANGERS.

Follow your instincts.

Your instincts are best verified by a quick Internet search, a call to the nurse line, or by referencing one of a dozen books written by dueling pediatricians or celebrities you didn't even know were mothers. Or, just trust the first online forum you find through Google.

Sharing a bed with your child helps you form an unbreakable bond that women for centuries and centuries have enjoyed.

Sharing a bed with your child is a great way to crush him in your sleep or KILL HIM WITH SIDS.

Putting your baby in his own room is cruel. What, are you going to let him *cry it out,* too? You know what crying is, right? It's a baby's natural reaction to wanting something because he can't express himself verbally. What kind of a mother would ignore that just so she can watch a few extra minutes of *Real Housewives*?

Crying it out is a great way to teach your child independence and resilience. Plus, I mean, babies cry. He'll get over it.

Nurse your baby in public, f*ck what all these uptight jackasses think of the female body. You're providing your child with the nutrients necessary for his development and survival.

This isn't *National Geographic,* put your nips away. How can I possibly explain to my children that you as a female have **breasts** and your child is eating from them? How can I possibly reconcile the fact that you are exercising your body's capability to nourish the life you brought into your world with the fact that I think of boobs as purely for my own sexual entertainment?

Formula is a perfectly safe alternative to breast milk. In fact, some scientists think it's better than breast milk, because it's made by science, unlike your boobs, which are just there for decoration.

Formula is great if you hate your baby. We're not judging at **all,** do what ya gotta do. But have you at least **tried** breastfeeding?

Savor every moment. Are you savoring the moment? Every. Single. Moment should be savored. Savor it. This moment. The moment that just passed. This upcoming moment. It's going to pass you by before you know it. You missed it. You should have savored it but you were busy reading this book or wondering when the next episode of *Property Brothers* is going to be on. *Property Brothers* is *always* on.

Go ahead and give him a bottle. You don't want him to starve while your milk comes in. Do you? Maybe you do and that's fine. You're the mother, after all.

Give him a bottle too soon and he'll reject your breast forever, opting instead to suckle from the sweet plastic teat you offered him too soon.

Every baby is different.

Every baby is different . . . buuuttttttt your baby should definitely be achieving certain milestones by a certain time. If he hasn't played the kazoo while using sign language to let you know he prefers a paraben-free lotion, I'm sorry but he is autistic.

But if he doesn't do that, I mean, no big deal. He's fine. Probably. Google it just to make sure.

Make sure your baby always has a hat on, because the heat is literally just shooting out of the top of his head at all times and you don't want him to get cold and die.

Make sure that there are no blankets in his bed, or he will die of SIDS.

Make sure your baby doesn't freeze to death in his crib, you monster.

His crib should be free of all bedding or bumpers, because, you know, SIDS.

Make sure he's not exposed to the slats of his crib or he'll get tangled up like a fish and die if SIDS doesn't get him first.

Your child should learn to soothe himself without the aid of a pacifier.

You are an absolute monster if you don't give him a pacifier; are you trying to raise a weak little thumb-sucking mama's boy?

Don't listen to any advice.

Follow your instincts.

(Or Google it.)

Chapter 29

Everyone Thinks Their Kid Is the Best but Mine Actually Is

Ralph Jay Purmort burst forth from my vagina on January 22, 2013. It was his due date, which is apparently rare, but I expected nothing less than punctuality and good manners from my offspring, so he slid on out at a decent hour, after not a ton of work, and he didn't tear my vagina apart in the process. He's a good guy.

Ralph showed up, was whisked off to the NICU, and four days later pulled a teeny-tiny version of *Prison Break*, trading the hundreds of cords and machines that had been hooked up to his little body for the freedom of living with his parents. He was not a cute baby. He was small and wormy, with a giant bruise on his head that looked like it was Voldemort trying to take human form. He'd had a bit of "trauma" coming through the "birth canal," which means he had bashed his head somewhere inside my vagina, and we were waiting for the swelling to go down. In the meantime, I double-filtered the Instagram photos and used creative cropping to make it look like he wasn't just a skinny, hairless, two-headed guinea pig.

Ralph was born just a few weeks after his father had his second brain surgery, to remove a pesky and persistent Stage IV glioblastoma brain tumor, which is a medical term for Totally Fucked. A week before Aaron tried—and failed—to catch Ralph as he sailed out of my lady parts, he had been lying in a hospital bed just a few floors away, confined to a room for forty-eight hours while a team of doctors and nurses pumped him full of poison, hoping to keep him alive by trying to kill the part of his body that was trying to kill him.

I know that every parent aside from mine believes their child to be special, but they are mistaken. My child, however, *is* special. Almost instantly, Ralph knew that he had not been born into a family where he would be the sun, worshiped and revolved around. He knew, inside that head with another head growing off of it that Aaron was the number-one priority in our household, followed closely by my trying to grow in my eyebrows after overplucking them as a high school junior.

The week before Ralph was born, when I was swollen with pride (and, as I found out a few days later, preeclampsia), Aaron's new chemo doctor (there might be a technical term for that) stopped in to meet us before his new treatment. I don't think she meant to recoil at the sight of me, but she did, twisting her face up in a way that indicated she had smelled something shitty, and that something was the baby growing inside of me.

"Oh," she said, clutching her clipboard to her chest, "you're pregnant." She ran her hand through her salt-and-pepper hair, cut short enough to show off the glass bead earrings I imagine she made herself, a way to blow off steam after long shifts walking through winding hallways of decaying patients, telling them the kind of thing she was about to tell me.

She went on to explain to me that what Aaron was doing was very serious, which I hadn't known before, you know, it being Stage IV cancer and all. I'd considered the past year of chemo and radiation to be our honeymoon, apparently. This new, very serious treatment would mean he would be very tired, and did I understand that? I nodded to show her that though I was clearly stupid, I was doing my best to comprehend the words coming out of her mouth. She went on to tell me that Aaron couldn't spend his time caring for a small baby, because he would be tired. He would be tired, because as she mentioned, the serious treatment would make him tired. It was serious. Aaron really needed to focus on himself, and that's why they (she) didn't usually recommend having babies.

As much as I appreciated being told I should basically consider giving up this child for adoption or throwing myself down a flight of stairs, I did what most adult women would do: I left the room to cry and make a phone call.

"Oh *God*," I sobbed to my big brother over the phone in the family waiting room, most likely loud enough for her to hear me, "now I'm worried that this baby is going to kill Aaron and it's all my fault."

My older brother, Austin, was used to picking up the phone to listen to several straight minutes of my ranting, so he waited patiently for me to take my first breath.

"Nora," he said, "babies aren't like that. They just . . . they kind of arrive and feel out the vibe of a family, and fill the need they see."

The women in our family only want to hear what they want to hear, and Austin's years of practice with two hysterical sisters had clearly paid off. I felt better.

I went back to Aaron's room, stopping at every nurses' station to let them rub my stomach, hoping Dr. Doom would see me.

Our first night at home as a family of three, Aaron and I were staring at a small, wrinkly little alien, asleep in a bassinet in the middle of our king-size bed. Ralph didn't make a single peep. I stayed up the entire night, to guard him from SIDS and ghosts, and I saw that my brother was right. This kid *got it*. He didn't cry or fuss when he was ready to eat, just turned his head toward me and opened his mouth, waiting for me to put a boob in it. He slept peacefully in a sling while I unloaded the dishwasher, made dinner, or played *Fruit Ninja* on our Xbox Kinect. Most babies have wild and uncontrollable limbs, but in Aaron's hospital bed, Ralph was always careful not to disturb his IV or kick the help button on the guardrail while he was cuddling. He let me nurse him in the MRI waiting room, and change his diaper in the Infusion Center, on one of those extra-wide waiting room chairs that at least ten thousand different butts have sat on. He happily cooed in the arms of the oncology nurses, who have spent more time with him than have some of his family members. One night, while Aaron and I were enjoying a typical hospital date night—takeout tacos in Styrofoam containers with *The Sopranos* streaming on a laptop— Ralph decided he wasn't happy at the foot of the hospital bed with his stuffed animals and pulled himself up to join us.

"He's crawling!" we shouted, ridiculously proud of the baby who was so lazy I had to take him to a special assessment at Children's Hospital just to be given "he's lazy" as an official diagnosis from a physical therapist. Before he could reach the laptop screen and the R-rated content of an HBO show, our room filled with nurses and nursing assistants, who cheered and scooped him up in their arms, whisking him down the hallway to celebrate his milestone while Aaron and I, beaming with pride, finished our dinner with Tony and Carmela.

Aaron and I were always a team. I'd never before loved someone who was always so definitively on my side (with the exception of the time he told me I couldn't make penny loafers cool, which I still disagree with and just attribute to the fact that his brain tumor was keeping him from seeing what a trendsetter I am). Ralph was the perfect addition to our little universe, and no matter what that doctor told me, I know for a fact that Ralph and his superior attitude are what kept Aaron alive for another year and a half. It's science.

After Ralph was born, when the nurses took him to the NICU and explained his issues to me in that vague horn noise the adults in *Peanuts* cartoons speak in, I lay alone in my hospital bed, in a pool of my own blood, and cried. Not because it hurt (the epidural kicked in riiiiiight at the end, so I felt pretty amazing) but because of what Aaron had said, after the baby slid through his hands and landed by my ankles.

"It's a boy!"

A boy. A boy who would spend his entire life being compared to his father, living in the shadow of a man he would barely get to know. It didn't help that beneath the wrinkles and baby acne and the peeling skin, Ralph did look exactly like Aaron. Which was also annoying, because I'd been the one who shared my Dairy Queen cones and Chipotle burritos with him for nine months. Me! And what do I get? His weird, overly flexible thumbs. That's *all*.

I worry about that less now. Children grow into who they will be, regardless of what they look like. That's how my sister turned out to be a forty-year-old white woman in a Bollywood dance troupe, and how my brother turned out to be a twenty-eight-year-old who collects cuckoo clocks and uses a cut of rope to hold his belt up. I won't be able to actually help it if Ralph grows up to be the kind of guy who grows white boy dreads; I can just hope I've given him the tools he needs to make better choices, and make sure he's excluded from my will if he makes such an infraction.

The day that Aaron died, I'd banished everyone from our house except the three of us. For weeks, our house had been filled with family, and we needed to be a unit again, our own little universe. Ralph was nearly two, which is a pretty terrible age unless, again, you are talking about my child. He walked quietly into the room where Aaron lay unconscious in a hospital bed. The same kind of bed we'd become secretly engaged in, the same kind of bed where Ralphie had learned to crawl. He carefully climbed up beside his father, without disturbing any of the cords, and gently laid his giant head next to Aaron's. "I luh you, Papa," he said, sucking his thumb and rubbing the top of his head. "Bye bye."

Losing Aaron was like having our sun burn out, but Ralph and I learned to revolve around each other. I get to watch him become the person he is, and he gets to watch me become a mother, though he still looks at me as though he's skeptical of my capabilities.

Like Aaron, Ralph is not amused by my singing or dancing. "Stop that!" he'll say, covering his ears and eyes when I try to change the lyrics to popular songs to reflect my unique personal take on motherhood.

Like me, Ralph knows all the best swear words and how to use them in context. "Slow down!" he'll shout at cars that race through our neighborhood. "We live here, jackass!"

And like only he can, he still understands that he was born into a different kind of family, that his normal is not like any other kid's normal. Someday, I'm sure, he'll tell his therapist about how having his childhood documented via hashtag (#ralphiegrams) ruined his life, but for now, he seems to be thriving in the chaos of our little universe. He quietly flies across the country with me, laying his head in my lap and elevating his crossed ankles on his armrest like he's kicking up after a hard day, then waking up for a snack and an episode of *Curious George* as we near landing. He is as happy at day care as he is spending the day at a winery in Sonoma, or driving through the Arizona desert. He is flexible and resilient, and the only routine he has is his nightly prayers: one for my father, one for Aaron.

"Mama," he says to me, smiling up from the tower of LEGOs he's assembled on our living room floor after we've returned from another trip, "you're a strong guy."

Chapter 30

Hoarder

My siblings and I are suddenly feral children. This would be more sympathetic if we were actual children, but we are all over the age of thirty, with offspring of our own.

Grief strips you skinless. Skin is important not just for looks, but because without it, you are just a walking pile of exposed nerve endings. That's really the only way to describe our family right now, a bunch of skinless freaks brushing up against our memories just to feel the pain.

This sucks because we used to be a lot of fun. It's pretty typical for my siblings and I to laugh so much at one another's jokes that 1) our dad used to threaten us with physical violence and/or 2) our significant others completely remove themselves from the situation and form their own social gathering in another room without us even noticing.

But lately, something has been off. Namely, our skin. And also, our vibe. We're awkward and strange around one another, our jokes are more pointed, and none of us has a sense of humor anymore. My brother has recently taken offense to us referring to his "serape" as a "shawl." I'm no longer entertained by any jokes about my loosey-goosey parenting. Actually, I'm just not entertained by anything at all, period.

My mother invited us all over for Sunday breakfast. We thought we'd make it a tradition, a way to make sure that our busy schedules always have time for us as a Family with a capital *F,* even if we are conspicuously two fewer every time we meet. Our children are playing in the "clubhouse," a big, light-filled room off my mother's kitchen that used to be a dark, one-stall garage and is now a page out of a Martha Stewart photo shoot, with floor-to-vaulted-ceiling bookshelves. She doesn't mind that her five grandchildren stand on her beautiful sofa and rub their greasy hands on the beautiful rug, so we let them govern themselves while my siblings and I sit around the dining room table and let our mother wait on us.

Our mother is standing over the griddle she's had since the eighties. It's made it to five different basements since then, where it's hauled out for occasions like this: when a skillet and a stove just can't keep pace with the kind of pancake consumption that's about to take place.

I woke up yesterday feeling more bruised than usual. I canceled all my plans. I gave away the tickets to the Sleater-Kinney concert that Aaron and I had bought for each other months before he died. They would be playing on Valentine's Day, their first tour in a decade or so. I drove my car through our city, haunted with memories, and cried so hard that when I stole a glance at the car next to me at a red light, they gave me the sort of tentative smile I imagine you'd give a total serial killer if he happened to pull up next to you.

But my siblings don't know that, because it's not the kind of thing you tend to exchange in a family text message.

My miscarriage, my father's death, my husband's death have all compounded inside me. It is grief on grief on grief. Grief to the third degree. It is grief, with interest. And that's not even taking into account their grief, because I am too selfish to care about that right now.

I had looked around the room in the ICU when our father was dying and felt a flood of gratitude for each of my siblings, followed by a flood of panic for my only son. The death of a parent is agonizing, but was made more bearable by each of them. Or maybe not more bearable. Not at all, actually. It was a comfort to have them, but grief is not a set weight to be distributed equally. It cannot be portioned and divided.

It's hard for me to be around my family—Aaron's family, too—and this is why. Grief is lonely, no matter how many other people feel it. They are different, each one, because we've lost different people, different versions of the same men. We are each carrying our own load, and it is ours alone to bear.

My siblings and I are all so busy licking our own wounds that we've forgotten how damaged we all are, so consumed are we by our own individual grief. We are trying, though, like a group of aliens trying to pass as humans by aping the behaviors we've observed in others. We hug hello, we try to laugh and joke the way we always have: at the expense of one of us. It is forced and awkward, and I know I should have stayed home today because I am not in a mood for pretending everything is okay when it is not.

Since I've arrived, thirty minutes late and unshowered, I've been sitting cross-legged at the table idly staring at my phone, mindlessly scrolling through feeds that show me what people I barely know are thinking and watching and eating, silencing my own thoughts like some terrible scene from a Ray Bradbury novel, half listening to anything. My siblings are arguing over our impending family vacation in early June, which my mother has arranged for us at a lodge in northern Wisconsin. My little brother, Patrick, is insisting that his family can't make it, and somehow he brings up the topic of our last family vacation.

Our family had never taken a vacation together, not all four children and both parents, not ever. But we gave it a go last summer, spending the week before Labor Day at an aging resort in northern Minnesota. It was cold and rainy most of the time, and Aaron lay in bed in the back of the A-frame cabin, my father across the hall, both of them pretending they weren't dying. They kept their toiletry bags side by side in the bathroom, and I knew next year that shelf would be empty, that neither of them would be here with us. My father and Aaron stuck it out on those rickety cabin beds and sofas as long as they could. We left for the city the morning after Patrick, his wife, and their baby finished their four-hour drive to the resort.

It must have been maddening for him, and exhausting for his baby. And disappointing. But right here? In this moment, just three months after the death of a husband who will never take another vacation with me again? I. Don't. Care.

I look up from my phone just long enough to tell him that: I don't care how disappointed he is with the last trip we took. We left because Aaron was dying, doesn't he get that? Doesn't he know that's the last trip I'll ever have with my husband, who would do anything to sit in a car and head up north again, even if just for a night?

I deliver this bitingly, though hardly looking up from my phone, where my pointer finger scrolls, scrolls, scrolls, the faces of old acquaintances and perfect strangers flying by while my brother pulls my daggers out of his chest.

I believe Elizabeth Kübler-Ross would call this the anger phase of grief, but in my heart I fear it is something worse: that without the spell of Aaron's love, the ugly Nora Beast I thought was gone has returned.

Even as a small child I was always easily wounded, quick to anger, and slow to let go of a grudge. My father always told the story of Leo French, some man who insulted my grandfather's suit during the Depression, a trespass so grave that my grandfather, delirious in his old age, would go on and on about "that damn Leo French."

"Let it go," my dad would say when I would rage on about any and all perceived slights from classmates, teachers, or siblings, "This is your Leo French."

Everything was my Leo French. (And Mr. French, if your ancestors are reading this, I hope they know you were a real bastard for insulting my prince of a grandfather.) When I was ten, I wrote entire diary entries about why I didn't love my mother. Among other failings, she always took my brother's side, never believed in me, didn't love me at all, and always took my brother's side. That final point was so important it was listed multiple times. I would scream and cry and throw tantrums so crazed that my family would just stare in disbelief at the rabid child before them and say, "Nora, don't throw a fit and fall in it," which most child psychologists agree is definitely the correct thing to say to a child dealing with complex emotions.

I had a lot of feelings as a child, and a lot of empathy. I'd cry sometimes, alone in my room, out of sadness for the old man with Parkinson's who seemed so embarrassed by his condition in mass. We always sat a few pews behind him, and as the months passed and the shaking became more apparent, he'd graduated from using his good arm to brace the wild one to just sitting on his shaking hand and I'd stare at the back of his head and say, "I love you," in my head like that had special healing powers. But I was also cruel and biting. Sometimes in ways I learned from watching cliques of cool girls form around me, and sometimes in ways I innovated myself. Maybe all children are like this: a tender little heart wrapped in barbed wire. I was a razor blade in an apple. If an apple was a taller, uglier fruit that wasn't as popular as an apple, but wanted to be. So, maybe a banana? Clever and well-read and ugly is the perfect combination if you're trying to make a Swiss Army knife of a girl with any number of ways to protect herself and cut a person down.

Time helped me to soften these sharp edges, to grow a shell that prevented me from absorbing every hurt, and prevented me from slicing into people without thinking twice. But Aaron's love and Aaron's sickness and Aaron's death had helped form me into a new person, a new Nora. Today I don't feel like the old Nora or the new one. I don't feel like Nora at all.

It is true that grief is lonely. It is true that nobody can do this for me, that I must grieve my grief alone. It is true that when you type the word "grief" this many times, it starts to lose its meaning completely and starts to look like it is always spelled wrong. But it is also true that grief cannot be measured, that I have assigned a higher value to my own sorrow than I have to that of the people who love me most, that I have allowed my own feelings to invalidate theirs. It is not a contest you can win: Who here has the most dead people? Me! I do! Because we all lost Aaron and our father but only I lost *her*. I'd decided—we'd decided, Aaron and I together—that it was a girl I was carrying. She felt different from Ralph right away, a little feminine force developing inside of me. I am the only one left here to mourn her, and I didn't get a chance to, not really, because my father and Aaron followed her so quickly into the everywhere.

I have never felt more tenderness for any of my siblings than I did on November 25, when each of them was there to hold me and Aaron, to hug his mother and his sister, to pour me a glass of wine and put my son to bed. I'd picked out everything for Aaron to wear to his cremation except his socks—a huge oversight for a man whose sock collection took up an entire bureau drawer—and my two brothers labored over this point with the same attention to detail that Aaron would have brought to the situation, holding different pairs of novelty socks up against his J.Crew button-down and sweater until they found the perfect complement. They folded his hands over his chest. They stayed in the room, their hands resting on his shoulders, as if he still needed comfort. That tenderness has calloused over, and today I cannot feel for anyone but myself and my own exposed nerves.

You know those episodes of *Hoarders* where they're trying to get a woman to let go of a room full of legit garbage and she's like, "I don't see the problem," while a stranger is literally shoveling out piles of dead cats and old magazines? That's me, collecting all my sorrows, mooning over my ghoulish collection, completely oblivious to the people around me who want to help shovel some of this shit out, or at least organize it into piles.

Here! I want to say. *Take it! The floor is about to cave in and I'm going to start peeing in a bucket at any moment!* But I can't say that, because we aren't talking anymore, any of us. My little brother packs up his diaper bag and zips his daughter into her snowsuit and leaves the house. My mother follows him outside. Nobody says another word to me, not for days, so I keep it all to myself.

Chapter 31

You're Doing a Good Job

Really, you are. I know it doesn't feel that way because everyone you know seems to be doing a better job at life than you are, but they're *not*. They're just really good at posting happy things to Facebook and Instagram.

You're doing a good job at work, even though your boss sends you douchey emails at 11:00 P.M. with entire paragraphs in the subject line and even though your coworkers do annoying things like cc'ing the whole team on emails in which they basically throw you under the bus, but use emoticons to lessen the feeling of the tires crushing your spine. Remember that work is just work, it's not your entire life. It's just a thing you do during the day that helps finance your real passion for sitting on the couch watching TV and eating string cheese. You're good at what you do—great, really—so if these clowns can't see that, you can just dust off the old résumé and find somewhere new to work.

You're doing a good job of being a parent, unless you're *not* a parent, in which case, if you ever choose to be a parent, you'll probably end up being pretty good at it, I'd guess. If you are a parent, like I said, you're doing a pretty good job! Sure, you may have carried your baby wrong, Ryan Reynolds, but big deal! Who doesn't do that?! Who has ever done parenting exactly right? Who hasn't accidentally hit their son's head on the car door while trying to wrestle him into a car seat? Who hasn't given her child a penny to keep him occupied, and then discovered he has stored it in his cheek for safekeeping? Big deal! Your kids are growing up to be fine, wonderful humans because you did or did not put them in baby yoga already and they already do or do not speak two languages. Statistically speaking, you only need to worry about them being a mass murderer or orchestrating the financial meltdown of our nation if you're raising a white male, so don't sweat it too much.

You're doing a good job at friendship, even if you unfollowed most of your friends on Facebook because they complained about having a cold as if they had just been diagnosed with incurable brain cancer, and even if you insist on making a huge deal out of your birthday after age twenty-one. I love you, but you do need to stop with the birthday shit, guys. I get that you're excited about being alive but nobody gets a birthday *month,* and your friends are only pretending to tolerate it. You were born like everyone else on this planet, so stop acting like you're the first one to do it. Just buy yourself something expensive that you don't need, post a thank-you for all the "HBD" wishes on Facebook, and then quietly lament the quick passing of your one precious life, like the rest of us.

You're doing a good job at being a grown-up, too. I know it doesn't feel like it because you recently overdrew your checking account and woke up hungover at 2:00 P.M. on a Sunday, but seriously, you are crushing it. I don't even know if people say "crushing it" anymore, but that's the only way to describe what you're doing. You've mostly paid your bills on time, you're in a reasonably good relationship or you're single because you just cannot be tamed right now, and you may or may not be a parent. Who is doing a better job at life than you are? The only person who comes to mind is my two-year-old son, and only because he can threaten to wipe his butt on me and somehow make it cute. Otherwise, you're probably tied for first place with him.

The only reason nobody else has told you how good of a job you're doing is because they're all so nervous *they're* not doing a good job that they can't even see what a good job you're doing. Just out of frame of those perfectly staged Instagram photos are the same piles of unopened mail and dirty dishes and the same crushing sense of doubt that's sitting on your chest right now, you just can't tell because of the filter. My personal fav is Valencia. It makes me look competent and hides my acne.

Being alive is really hard sometimes, and all we want is a little bit of credit. So here: As long as you never offer to take me to lunch and then try to recruit me for your pyramid scheme—I'm sorry—*network marketing opportunity,* trust me, you're doing a good job.

Chapter 32

Relationship Porn (XXX, NSFW)

FANTASY SCENARIOS FOR THE CHRONICALLY LONELY

You and your partner, on the couch, watching a *Game of Thrones* marathon. He turns to you and calls you his Khaleesi. You both ignore that Khal Drogo had a really fucked-up death.

A man wearing a wedding ring, a little symbol that he is proud to belong to somebody.

You see two people walking down the street holding hands. Their steps fall in perfect unison without their even trying.

A couple is sitting in a crowded restaurant having a face-to-face conversation. They laugh and order dessert. They never pick up their phones.

Your lady friend is picking up takeout on the way home because she knows you have to work late and she wants you to have one less thing to worry about.

Your boyfriend plays with the ends of your hair while you watch a movie. The movie is whatever you wanted to watch.

You can't decide between the burger or the Caesar salad. You get the salad but your partner gets the burger. "We'll split them!" you say. You eat a third of his burger and most of his fries and all of your salad.

Your wife, lying next to you in bed, reading while wearing the retainer she got when she was thirteen.

Your partner buys concert tickets for both of you without even asking if you want to see the show. You're not crazy about the band, but you go anyway.

It's garbage day and your husband said he'd take the garbage out last night, but he didn't, so it's still in the driveway and now you have to wait until next week. You send him a passive-aggressive "what day is garbage?" text before you leave for work. You know what day garbage is.

Your girlfriend texts to ask if you guys need dental floss, because she's at Target and could pick some up.

Your husband makes dinner, feeds the baby, cleans up the entire kitchen, and puts the kids to bed while you paint your nails and watch *Gilmore Girls* reruns.

You and your friends are standing in the back of a concert talking and your boyfriend gets each of you a beer on his way back from the bathroom.

You ask your wife what she wants for dinner. She says, "I don't know, probably just a bowl of cereal?" And you sit on the couch eating a box of Lucky Charms together because you are adults.

You look fly as hell and your partner takes your photo for Instagram so you don't need to post a mirror selfie.

The baby is up at 7:00 A.M. on a Saturday, which is rude because you have a hangover. Your partner says, "I'll get him. You keep sleeping."

Your boyfriend left the cap off the toothpaste again. You're like, "Dude, you *need* to put the cap on the toothpaste! It's all dried out now!" And throw it dramatically in the garbage. He apologizes.

You check your phone in the middle of the workday. Your person has sent you a text. He wants to know how your day is. He's just taking a second to say hello to his person, and his person is you.

Chapter 33

Cool Widow Kind of Wants to Kiss Someone

WARNING: This whole part is about sex so if you are related to me, you'll probably want to skip it. If this sounds prudish, that's because I guess I'm still a bit of a prude. Once I thought I heard my dad making sex noises at night, and when I brought it up, indignantly, to my mother the next morning, I was relieved to find out he was having Vietnam flashbacks in his sleep. There are a lot of things wrong with that, I know.

I started dreaming about sex the month after Aaron died, waking up hot and lonely and very uncomfortable about the things I'd dreamed of doing with the guy from the food co-op who always sighs with disappointment when I say no, I am not a member, before he swipes my credit card. A little guilty, too, to be so corporeal, so tied up in my living body that I could find the time to feel something like that when Aaron's death is so fresh. But I felt it. I feel it all the time. Even though my battered heart is barely beating, even though I've got no capacity to possibly add another human to the list of people I love, my body is craving connection.

"Well, I'm on Match.com," I started telling my friends, around the same time. Not because I was, but because I wanted to see their reactions. They were all the same: the same uncomfortable smiles and nods, the same high-pitched "Okay! Good for you!" and the same relieved laughter when I told them I was joking.

But I don't know why exactly I'm saying that as a joke. It's not particularly funny, and it's not particularly outlandish. I mean, I'm thirty-two. I haven't had sex for the last time. Right?

When Aaron was still alive, one of my first widow friends texted me to say that she had started online dating.

"Good for you!" I texted, but inside I recoiled in horror. It had been four months since her husband died. *Four months.* Surely, I thought, wrapping my arms around my living husband's ever-diminishing waist, it takes longer than that to heal from such a loss.

And yep, it does.

But we're not talking about healing. And we're not talking about falling in love. We're talking about sex. Or, like, honestly, at this point, just hugging or kissing. Or just someone to play with my hair. Or even someone who would just put his hand on the small of my back while we're walking into a restaurant. Also, someone to pay for dinner and listen to my stories and laugh wholeheartedly and tell me that I'm funny. Also, somebody who doesn't know me and pity me, the poor widowed mother, who has just *been through so much.*

I am a thirty-two-year-old woman who has not been touched by a man in many months. I have not gone this long without male contact since losing my virginity, which I held on to for nearly twenty years, to the horror of my high school self, who had promised to wait until marriage, though what the hell did that girl know? She pierced her belly button as a direct result of seeing Britney Spears with a belly ring on *Total Request Live*.

Anyway, it has been a while and I am finding my hunger is coming out in new ways. I sometimes hug my male friends a little too long. The other day, a CrossFit coach gently brushed my shoulder while adjusting my form and I swear I had an orgasm.

I. Am. Lonely.

I've been alone—and lonely—before, though they aren't the same thing.

Taylor Swift is alone. Well, actually, she started seeing Calvin Harris, as I write this, and I'm weirdly jealous, like we'd both agreed to go to prom alone and then she showed up with a date or something. But even when Taylor is alone, she's not *lonely*. She's amassing a huge collection of supermodel best friends and baking pies and making hits. And that's what I'm doing, basically! Except it's more like parenting a child and buying gluten-free cookies and watching *Scandal* on the couch with my friends. And except that I want my own Calvin Harris. At least for a night or two.

At four months of widowhood, my friends understand. Or some of them do. The more prudish ones, who, like me, probably leave the room during sex scenes when they're watching movies with their family, are uncomfortable with my need. "Nora," they say about my desire to casually kiss a man, a fairly innocent affair by even the most prudish of standards, "it will just be like junk food. Totally empty calories and completely unsatisfying." These are people who have never been this kind of lonely. And who probably don't eat pints of gelato for dinner.

This is not a normal kind of lonely. This is a new brand of loneliness for me. I am lonely the way any person without a partner is lonely, the way that old men buying only canned soup and Oreo cookies in grocery stores are lonely. It's being lonely for the marriage we had and the life we shared together, where I got to text "On my way" when I left the office and had someone to send me new pop sensations before they hit the radio. It's a loneliness for the simple feeling of belonging to someone, or having that person belong to me, like the rings we wore on our left hands, a little signal to the world that we were someone's person.

I am a really fun person to be around right now, as you can imagine.

I want an out, I want a lifeline. I want that lifeline to be a very handsome stranger who thinks I am very cool and basically loves me but knows I am a loner and a rebel right now, someone who wants into the little clubhouse I've built with Ralph but understands that he must wait to be invited before crossing the threshold, like a vampire.

I want someone who is kind and loving, but won't love me, or expect me to love him. Just someone who thinks I am fantastic and wants to kiss me and maybe hug me, who respects me but also doesn't want anything from me. I basically want a male escort who only kisses and also assembles IKEA furniture and kills spiders.

It's been over four years since I've been on a date, and I'm finding, like people find out when they're released from prison after thirty years, that the world has changed. There are electric cars! Nobody says "raise the roof" anymore! We can shop for humans using our cell phones!

I'm not sure if the "game" ever involved recent widows just seeking a person to physically touch them without expecting a relationship or even sex, but the closest thing I can find to such a request that doesn't involve the risk of becoming a Craigslist-killer victim is, I guess, Tinder.

For those of you who have never had to use Tinder because you've been in a happy adult relationship since before 2014, GOOD

FOR YOU, TREASURE THE PERSON WHO LOVES YOU FOR
SAVING YOU FROM THIS HELL. Also, here is how it works:
You're served up some people who are currently in proximity to
you and also fit the gender you're seeking. If you like them, based
on their photos and bio, you swipe right. If you don't, you swipe
left. If you both like each other, you can send a message, eventually
meeting in person and kissing on the lips if you would like to.

Tinder is allegedly more anonymous than other dating apps
because there's no profile for people to search. I'm not on those
ones because it doesn't feel right to put myself in a dating pool
where boys from high school may be fishing for their second wife.
No, I need something with the reputation of a hook-up site, even if
what I'm looking for is decidedly PG.

I don't want to run the risk of being matched with anyone I
know, so I decide to test the waters when I'm visiting the Bay area
for a few weeks to work on this book. Surely I'll be able to find
someone tall, nerdy, and looking for a no-strings-attached above-
the-belt-only fling with a recent widow. Right?

First things first, I need a bio. Something to the point, but
intriguing.

NORA, 32.

About Nora:

A cool widow who kind of wants to kiss someone.

   In the Bay Area for a few weeks, hanging out and writing a
book (BRAG). I am very tall (6'), and I also have a toddler who
you won't ever meet because I'm not a crazy person. I just want
to be around a live adult male and maybe kiss him. MAYBE.

I always include my height in any description of myself, because
I'm incredibly tall for any human, but especially for a woman, and
I want people to be prepared for what they're going to encounter. I

personally don't care anymore when complete strangers do double takes when spotting me in the wild, or men I've never met insist on going back-to-back to see who is taller (me, always). I just want to spare fragile males the discomfort of trying to explain to me that they are six feet tall and I must be taller than I think I am.

Once my profile is up, I can start shopping. There's not actually information about how tall a person is, and most men seem to be completely inept at choosing appealing photos of themselves that don't include other people's children or a fish they caught.

I'm trying to be open-minded, but it's really hard to discern whether someone has the qualities I'm looking for from just a few blurry photos and a few lines of copy where they indicate that they are, like every other man on Tinder, a nice guy who likes to eat food and do stuff.

Finally, I get a message.

> Hello Nora and welcome to the Bay Area! I loved your description!
> I share the same feeling of being around an adult woman and
> laugh and laugh and be serious and laugh again
> And eventually kiss.
> I know the toddler feeling as well.

I'm not sure what to do with this conversation, so I let it sit there in my inbox and hope this guy moves on to another adult woman who can laugh and be serious and laugh again. I do, however, wonder about his toddler feeling.

My second suitor pops up a day later.

> There's no way this is a real profile, but I at least want the name
> of the model you stole these photos from ;-)

I halfheartedly consider a few witty responses, but can't bring myself to reply. I don't know how I expected this to work, but this isn't it. I've heard Tinder described as the gamification of dating, but I don't really get that, because it's a boring-ass game. Swipe left, swipe right, and perhaps you will get a semi-literate message from a stranger with a few grainy photos! I'd rather just make eye contact with a bunch of strangers and then stalk through Craigslist "Missed Connections" looking for a description of a tall blonde with eyes like a starved wolf. I find the gear icon in the upper right-hand side of my screen and delete my profile.

It's been four months since Aaron died. That same widow friend I mentioned is still single, having found that the gnawing loneliness she was trying to satisfy won't be filled by someone served to us by an algorithm and a smartphone, won't be filled by sex at all.

This isn't something that you get over, it's just a gaping wound that I will learn to live with. Someday, I know, I will meet a man and I will love him. He will love me back, even though I never fully replace the caps on full containers of salad dressing or Tylenol. Even though I pee with the door a little bit open because I am lazy and even though I can't watch anything suspenseful without providing a running commentary for the sake of my own stress relief. I'll love him for all his weirdo traits, too, but I'll love him around the hole that Aaron left. Some spaces are not meant to be filled.

Chapter 34

Frenching in a Van

"Okay, if you want to make out with me you have exactly five minutes."

It's 11:55 P.M. and I'm in a van parked in front of my house with a guy I've been introduced to through Twitter. I've been stifling yawns—or not stifling them—for at least two hours. What does it take to get a man to just get down to business these days?

I haven't kissed someone—not like this—in months, and I'm not entirely sure how you do it. "Oh, are you going left?" I say, which is just the kind of dirty talk a man wants to hear while you close your eyes and move your mouth around like a starving baby bird. It turns out that kissing is like riding a bike in that I'm still not feeling coordinated enough to pull it off, but I'm somehow doing a fairly competent job at it. Also, I should be wearing a helmet.

I've had even more of a tendency toward self-absorption lately. There's something about having your spouse die and then quitting your job to freelance from home that makes you just a tad socially awkward. But I've been working on my social skills, and I know it's good to ask people about themselves instead of just talking about yourself, so I started this date out on a confident foot by asking my date a question.

"So," I said, buckling up as his van ambled its way down my street on a sunny spring evening, "tell me about your divorce!"

I realize, as a widowed mother over thirty living in the Midwest, that divorcés are going to be my lot in life moving forward. By thirty-five, an unmarried Midwestern man is clearly defective. But a divorced thirty-five-year-old man in the Midwest? He's just shaking off the mistakes of a wholesome youth where you believe, at twenty-two, that you should for sure marry that girl you'd like to have sex with someday.

Divorce is somewhat fascinating to me. Before my father died, my parents were married for forty years, and none of my friends growing up had divorced parents. Divorce always seemed dramatic and a bit scandalous, the kind of thing that happened on the TGIF shows I wasn't allowed to watch.

I've never been great at breakups, so I can't imagine how terrible I'd be at divorce. Wait, yes, I can. I have an excellent imagination. I'd demand we sign the papers in person, with fountain pens, and make a joint announcement through social media referring to it as a conscious uncoupling and asking our friends and family to respect our privacy. Then, I'd start vaguebooking about how "sometimes, you need to burn in the fires of betrayal to become the phoenix you are meant to be." Or, "Making like Taylor Swift and shaking it off! :-)." When the divorce was finalized, I'd insist on releasing burning paper lanterns into the air to symbolize the destruction of our once hopeful union, preferably within the presence of our new lovers, to really bring things full circle.

Instead, I completed my vows to the letter. I found someone who loved and understood me deeply, even when I was being bat-shit insane and saying things like "I found a centipede downstairs! Grab the baby, I'm going to burn this house to the ground!" My baggage isn't about someone not growing with me, or not choosing the same direction in life. It's not even baggage, really. It's a privilege to carry Aaron with me, and the right man is going to love me—and all the parts of me I got from loving Aaron. That man is probably not my date this evening, with his man bun and his vegetarian diet and his urge to sow the wild oats that I was busy sowing in my twenties while he was being someone's husband. But Manbun is so sweet and nice that he can be right for right now, I suppose.

I feel a small amount of shame for being out tonight, with a man who is not a friend, but a guy I'd sourced through Twitter for the sole purpose of satisfying my PG-13 sexual needs.

Where can a widow find a guy to make out with her? Asking for @noraborealis, my sister tweeted one night from my couch after a few glasses of white wine. Manbun was the clear front-runner for this job because he was the only person who replied, and he also came with references, having had a brief post-divorce fling with my friend Kelly, who described him as "passionate and willing to work hard between the sheets." In my twenties, I prided myself on being unable to produce a sexual Venn diagram with any of my friends, but I am no longer in my twenties. I am, as my nephew recently said, "young, but not really young . . . youngish." The last time I kissed a person romantically, he was dying. So when Manbun slid into my Twitter Direct Messages and offered up his phone number, I thought, what the hell, and texted him. I'd been spending a bit too much time trading flirtatious text messages with a friend who didn't let the fact that he had a girlfriend hold him back from texting me at all hours of the night.

Manbun is funny and clever and very cute. He knows everything about me already, because Google, but he still tries to get to know me.

I'd planned to just enjoy him through the glow of my iPhone, but something small shifted inside me. I'd attached so much meaning to the idea of my first kiss after Aaron. It's normal, I'm guessing, to have high expectations when the last romantic kiss you shared was on your beloved's deathbed. You're not just going to kiss any geek off the streets after that.

Manbun let me know that he wasn't really in a relationship space, but was down for a FWB situation, which I had to decipher using Google. He was just too busy for a real relationship, to which I replied that being a single mother didn't leave me with much free time and that also my heart was cold and dead and I wasn't looking for a boyfriend, either.

I wasn't going to fall in love with this guy, I knew, but I could at least let him take me out to drink and eat and hang out among other alive humans in our age bracket. What could be wrong with letting him put his hand on my knee after three drinks, or feeling the thrill of kissing a strange new mouth under a strange new beard that ended up not being strange at all. His beard feels just like Aaron's. He has the same heavy bottom lip and crooked teeth. He kisses me until his man bun comes undone, and I can feel myself coming alive again in my swimsuit zone. I notice, because I am the kind of person who keeps her eyes open when she's dry-humping in a family van in a residential neighborhood, that the digital clock has struck midnight.

"Okay! Time's up!" I say, and he lays his head, exasperated, on the soft curve of my exposed belly while I contemplate how I got here: a thirty-two-year-old woman Frenching in the front seat of a Honda Odyssey in front of the house where her mother is babysitting her two-year-old son.

The next day, I don't feel like I thought I'd feel: guilty and wrong.

I feel like I felt the day I took off my wedding ring, like the moment lacked the meaning I had anticipated it having.

I slid off my plain white-gold wedding band two days after Aaron's funeral, up north on the edge of Lake Superior for our annual anniversary trip to Grand Marais, an itty-bitty town that seems like it's perched at the edge of the earth. Since our last visit, a new store had sprouted up, filled with reimagined secondhand clothing and handmade jewelry. If Aaron were here, he'd buy me whatever I wanted. Not because we are rich, but because he was generous even with money that we didn't have. One of the women in this shop had created delicate little rings out of silver and pieces of glass that had been tumbled into opacity by the waves of Lake Superior. I slid my wedding band into my wallet for safekeeping as I tried on ring after ring after ring. None of them fit correctly, and my toddler was busy trying to destroy the entire shop with his own two hands, so I left empty-handed.

The next day, my left thumb brushed against my ring finger, absentmindedly searching for that plain white-gold band, which I'd spent three years spinning endlessly around my ring finger. It was still in my wallet, but I didn't reach for it. It was better, I knew, for it not to be a Thing with a capital *T,* another Big Event in a series of Big Fucking Events. It was better to have it just be something that happened quietly, without me even noticing.

So it's okay that the first guy I kissed after the love of my life is not the second love of my life. It is okay that I didn't feel butterflies the first moment that I saw him, and that I woke up the next morning and went about my life as usual, with no obsessive replay of the night before, or wondering how long I should wait to text him, with none of the hallmark behaviors of modern-day courtship even crossing my mind. It is perfectly fine to pine for the man I lost and long for the thrill of a man I have not yet met. It is okay to have all of these feelings, even in one single day, and then to take them all back. I don't have a heart to give away, so there is no pretending I do.

Five months after Aaron's funeral, the semipermanent depression my wedding ring had left in the flesh of my ring finger is gone and I have kissed one man. I still find myself spinning my invisible ring some days. I'm always surprised to realize it isn't there.

Chapter 35

How You Do It

"I don't know how you do it," people say. "I wouldn't be able to get out of bed in the morning." It's meant as a compliment—I must be so strong!—and it's nice to hear that people may think of me that way, but it's not exactly true.

I'm not stronger than anybody. I mean, physically, I can do three pull-ups, so I'm stronger than *some* people, but emotionally, I'm the same as anyone else. This strength isn't superhuman. It's the most human thing of all, a muscle we're all born with but need to exercise rarely at best. And lucky for us, it's a tenacious little thing that bounces back from atrophy as soon as you need to flex it.

While we're talking about muscles, yes, I do work out (thanks for asking). At one of those gyms that is filled with giant, heavy weights and ultra-fit humans and not much else. Working out is hard for me, probably because I am naturally lazy and like to take the easy way out. Sometimes, I'll skip a round if I have lunch plans after class and don't want to sweat too much. If I can't get in a full set of push-ups, I cut myself a break. One day, while I was complaining about how heavy the kettlebells were, my coach agreed with me. This workout was hard. "That's the thing," he said, "to get stronger, things have to get harder."

Both my shoulders and my inner strength are more developed now than they were a few years ago, because even though I try to half-ass it through push-ups and I got through most of my life with zero problems, I've been through some shit. And someday, you will, too. Maybe you won't lift weights—although it is recommended to keep our bone density up, ladies—but something hard is going to happen to you. Your husband may get sick. Your parents have a 100 percent chance of dying. I don't mean this as a scare tactic. I mean it as a pep talk.

Someday, the universe will throw a wrench in the works and your well-oiled machine of a life will grind to a halt. And then it will keep going. Because after you got bored of crying and worrying, you took a deep breath and pushed it back into motion.

"I don't know how you do it," someone will say to you while softly touching your arm.

But you'll know it's really nothing special to keep one foot moving after the other. You do it reflexively, like breathing, because it's not something you can choose not to do. The world goes on, even when you wish it would just lay on the bathroom floor with you for a little while. Your water bill still needs to be paid, they are adding your favorite shows from the nineties to Netflix, and your child insists on waking up and eating breakfast. Every. Day.

So, you do what needs to be done. You get through it. The way Britney got through 2007 and made it a distant memory and an Internet meme; the way Reese Witherspoon got through her divorce with Ryan Phillippe when he was super hot and now you're, like, Ryan *who*? The way Jackie Kennedy got through picking up pieces of her husband's brain and then married a Greek bajillionaire. The way Beyoncé got through the dismantling of Destiny's Child and emerged as *Beyoncé*. The way Khaleesi emerged from the fire and became the Mother of Dragons.

You won't do it because you are Superwoman, you'll do it because it's your life, and there is nobody who can live it for you. You will do it because you come from a long line of strong women. Women like Britney and Reese and Jackie. Women like Beyoncé. Women like your mom, who pushed you out of her vagina or picked you out of the whole world to love you and raise you up. Women like *you*, unless you are a man, in which case just imagine a woman you admire and be like her.

It was the middle of a normal Monday when Aaron had a seizure that turned out to be a brain tumor that turned out to be brain cancer that turned out to kill him. I'd woken up a normal twenty-seven-year-old woman who still had her hangover from Saturday night, and somewhere along the way, my life had been tilted on its side without my permission. I was not pleased. I had a very important PowerPoint to finish! I worked in advertising! I needed people to click on Internet ads and buy things! I made my mother drive me to the hospital, and I could feel my heart beating through my chest the entire three-mile ride from downtown to south Minneapolis. My mother had things to do at work, so she pulled up to the emergency room, leaned over me to open the door and all but pushed me out of the car.

"Go in there and be a woman," she said, and even though I had no idea what she meant, I did it.

Chapter 36

Please Like Me

Don't try to win over the haters,
you're not the jackass whisperer.
—BRENÉ BROWN

When I was ten, I ate dog biscuits because my friend told me to. As an adult, I can say something logical like, "Well, any girl who wants you to eat dog biscuits clearly isn't your friend," but Erica turned out to be a really good friend once she stopped making me eat dog biscuits after school for her own entertainment. Erica also gave me an ice cream cone to reward me for the dog biscuit I ate, so it's not like she was a total psycho. But even better: she liked me. I was in. We were going to be friends for life, because when she told me to eat a dog biscuit if I wanted an ice cream cone, I said yes and started chewing.

I would love to say that my dog biscuit days are over, and that I am one of those incredibly confident women who just doesn't care if you like her. Women on that list include Beyoncé and my mother and of course, Erica, who I liked immensely even while I was choking on a dog biscuit, and who grew up to be a pediatric intensive care nurse and real-life angel. It does not include me, because I am the human equivalent of a golden Lab. I just want your approval, even if I don't really like you and can smell that you are probably evil inside.

The Internet is a really great place to hone this skill. There, millions of people who are actually strangers who have never met you at all can say whatever they please about you. And even though I know in my heart that nothing good ever comes from entering the comments section, I occasionally take a peek. And it doesn't matter how many nice people say nice things about you, because you know from your middle school days that you don't remember them. No, what you remember is the stranger who described you as "just awful" and the girl at a sleepover who told you that you would be pretty if it weren't for your face. In both instances, my reaction should be, "Well, okay, fuck you, too," but instead it is something more like, "But, okay, how can I change myself to make you like me and what can I do to earn your approval? Because I'll do it, stranger. I will change everything about me to get you to like me, even though we will never meet in person, and your comments should have no bearing on my actual life."

An obsessive need to be liked is problematic. First, it's not very practical. You're not going to get everyone to like you, even if you're a wonderful human. I once saw a kid give a nun the middle finger, and you're (probably) not a nun. And to paraphrase Brené Brown, trying to get everyone to like you is time-consuming and exhausting, and it will take up the free time you could be spending with the people who don't need convincing that you are excellent.

I know that sounds like something your mom would say, but I'm a mom, and your mom and I are right.

I live every day with a reminder of how dumb it is to try to convince someone to like you. I only see it about three times a week because I don't shower that often, but on my back is a tattoo. A dumb one that means nothing and wasn't particularly well done by the guy in Brooklyn who was telling me about his hangover while etching an indelible vector image across my ribs. I don't want to get into the details about what the tattoo is specifically, but if you were imagining a circle of barbed wire around a four-leaf clover, right over a Chinese symbol for strength? You're wrong. But close.

Tale as old as time: I got this stupid-ass tattoo to impress a girl. I met Ricky when I met all my other Brooklyn roommates, at a party. I had a boyfriend at the time, and we were cohabitating in Queens. It was shaping up to be the saddest, loneliest year of my life, but finally he let me tag along with him to a party, and then I met Lauren. Lauren was very cool and thin and covered in layers and layers of vintage jewelry, like an Olsen twin. She was standing on her deck chain-smoking Parliament Lights while I chugged beer after beer and stood alone, trying to figure out what to do with my hands. Between drags, Lauren asked me where I lived, and with who. When I pointed out my boyfriend, she shook her head. "Nope," she said, "we're too young for that shit. Move in with us." Us? I was going to be a part of an "us"?? Us was two other girls: sweet Lorraine, who baked and sewed and was beautiful inside and out . . . and Ricky.

Ricky was instantly terrifying and magnetic. For one, she had a tattoo of her name on her bicep, and hair that was dyed jet black. She said "fuck" a lot, even by my standards, and she had a way of sort of looking just beyond you while you were talking.

I wanted her to love me, and she did. Until we actually all moved in together, when Ricky decided she hated me for things like being in the kitchen when she wanted to be in the kitchen, buying food that was similar to hers, cooking too much or too infrequently in our shared kitchen, or having friends over on a Sunday, which was the day she used to spend three hours in the bathroom on an exhaustive beauty routine, the details of which we could only guess at but which seemed to require a whole lot of concentration. In between hating me, she would sometimes decide to like me for brief, sparkling moments of time. She'd stand near me at a bar and not turn her back to me, she'd put me on a funny email chain, she'd sit down on the couch and watch some VH1 reality shows with me and not say anything mean to me. It was awesome.

During the years—yes, years—that we lived together, tattoos were really hitting the mainstream. I know that's a dorky thing to say, but this was right when Amy Winehouse was getting big, and full-sleeve tattoos went from being a sign that you were comfortable on the outskirts of society to being the kind of thing that fat suburban dads in cargo pants proudly sported. So one day, when Ricky made an appointment for a new tattoo, I went with her. "Really?" she said, and I sensed in her a very, very faint interest in me as a person. "Yeah," I lied, "I've been thinking about it forever so I think it's time."

Ricky doted on me for the whole week after I mangled my torso. She brought me ice packs and spread Aquaphor across my back to speed the healing process. And then, just as quickly, she was done with me. I think because I once had my boyfriend over at the apartment where I paid rent, and he went pee in the bathroom at some point and she didn't like that.

Ricky and I moved out of the apartment and we never spoke again. But I have a permanent memento of our time together. It's not quite as bad as getting a tattoo that says "no regrats" but the sentiment is the same. The tattoo isn't the worst thing I've done to get someone to like me—I did eat dog biscuits, and started smoking, and pretended to be interested in hockey—but it's the most permanent. And while that's a very valuable lesson and a good story for my children to hear someday, this tattoo has got to go.

Like most mistakes, it is easy come and long, grueling go. Instead of the instant gratification you get when you get a tattoo, you have one appointment every six weeks, where you feel like your skin is being hammered with a million tiny nails, and afterward, things look slightly different.

When it is gone, my skin will still have a little bit of scarring, because the tattoo wasn't really done correctly and because that happens sometimes when you try to undo a permanent change to your body. I'm okay with that. Things change, and so do people.

I can't do everything right, and I can't make everyone like me. And Lord knows I can't erase most of the mistakes of my twenties. But I can start with this one.

Chapter 37

I Don't Want to
Make It Look Easy

As humans in a Western society that prizes efficiency and resiliency and general get-the-fuck-over-it-ness, I'm afraid that I'm contributing to the notion that happiness is just about pulling yourself up by the bootstraps and taking a deep breath when life delivers a Chuck Norris throat punch right to your esophagus.

"You make it look easy," my sister told me one day while I fell apart in the front seat of her car, wiping my nose on my jacket sleeve and rambling incoherently about how nobody gets it, and everybody thinks I'm totally fine when I can't hear that Wiz Khalifa song from *Furious 7* without crying over my dad and Aaron and Paul Walker.

It's easy to make it look easy because I learned from the best. I complained more about my period than Aaron ever did about having brain cancer. Even when the tumor was pushing through new parts of his brain, shutting down his left arm and eventually his left leg, he was really chill. He laughed and smiled and made me stay up later than 10:00 P.M. watching *Buffy* on Netflix. It wasn't easy, I know. I was there to see him sleep twenty hours a day, to help button his shirts for him, to hold Ralph up to his face for hugs and kisses when he could no longer lift him. If he never felt sorry for himself, how could I feel sorry for me?

The thing is, it *is* easier for me than it is for some people. I know that even though I miscarried a baby and my dad and husband died a few weeks later, I'm a privileged person. Even grief is a privilege. Some women don't get to quit their jobs and write a book when their lives explode, they just have to turn up to work the next day and hope they find the time to pick up the pieces of their old lives at a later date.

Grief is weird, guys. Most books talk about it in nature terms, like it is a churning ocean, with waves and riptides and eddies that can pull you under. But mine is more like an expert stalker, adept at sneaking up on me undetected and strangling me from behind. He's too slick for most people even to notice, but he's there in the shadows, lurking at the edge of my happy Instagram photos, waiting to choke me out.

People *want* me to grieve. Sort of. They want me to be sad, but not so sad that I get drunk and cry at a stylish bar downtown. They want me to be happy, but not so happy that I go on a date with a man in public and maybe let him kiss me. They want me to move on, but not too quickly, and with one eye trained on the rearview mirror. They want me to grieve, but they don't want me to be a downer. Like, be mostly happy and, if it's not too much to ask, compartmentalize and schedule my grief for convenient times, like, perhaps from 7:00 to 9:00 P.M. on Monday, Wednesday, and Friday evenings.

"Be kind," we post on Facebook, "for everyone you meet is facing a hard battle." We attribute that quote to everyone from Aristotle to Marilyn Monroe, and then we go about our business doing our best not to look at the hard things. Unless they're already over, in which case they're not a hard thing anymore, they're an obstacle overcome, an enemy vanquished. Now it's a success story with a happy ending! People want it to look easy. And I don't blame them, because it's exhausting to watch someone struggle. Ask Lindsay Lohan. People don't want to see you falling out of a cab without your underpants on, they want to see you pretending to be twins who want their parents to get back together.

I had a habit of always, always choosing the subway car that would inevitably serve as a makeshift theater for a doo-wop band, an evangelist from the Deep South who believes he will make a difference in the world by screaming about sin in a crowded train, or a run-of-the-mill panhandler.

But one day, the crowds parted as if they'd seen a leper. Close enough. It was a man who was so badly burned his face was little more than a skull with a thin layer of pink skin, rippled and ridged, stretched tight across. I only knew he was a man because his beat-up cardboard sign held photos of him before his accident, smiling and normal, with all his facial features. He didn't say a word, just jangled the coffee can he used to collect money as he made his way through the car. I didn't have any money with me, because I prefer to deal only in the imaginary funds of credit cards, but when he made his way to my end of the car, I temporarily broke my concentration on the idiotic matching game I'd been laboring over for months and looked him in the eye.

"I'm sorry," I said. I meant because I didn't have any money. And because this was the shitty deal he got out of life: shuffling through train cars begging for cash from strangers who didn't want to see him.

I have it easier than a guy who got his face burned off and now begs for pennies on the F train, I know that. My life is hard, but just being alive can be hard. Even I need a reminder of that, especially when people on Facebook are complaining about seasonal allergies like they were just diagnosed with a terminal form of cancer. It's harder than it looks for everyone.

If you ask me how I am, I'll tell you reflexively that I'm okay. And it's true, for the most part.

And when you tell me the same thing, I'll know that it's mostly true for you, too. Because you're working hard to be that way. Not because it's easy.

Chapter 38

No

Because my son is a walking cliché of a toddler, he loves Curious George, bananas, and saying no. He says it even when he means yes, like when I ask if he has pooped his pants or if he needs a nap or if he likes ice cream. No, no, no.

He's persistent and predictable and damn it, he is wise. No gets harder to say the older we get. We are too encumbered by the expectations of other people to offer them just those two letters as a reply. Instead, we say:

"I'd love to, but . . ."

"Oh, I can't right now, but . . ."

"Actually, I'd just rather not . . ."

No is good. No is valuable. I know all those articles people share on Facebook are all about "Seven reasons to say YES TO EVERY-THING!" But they are a lie. No was invented to protect us from ourselves and our natural inclination to want to be agreeable, to be like the Facebook posts that insist we should embrace everything with a nod and a smile.

No has your back. No prevents you from going on three dates with a guy you are barely interested in, and suddenly finding yourself in a year-long relationship because you didn't want to hurt his feelings and tell him you weren't interested after you watched him eat spaghetti.

No keeps you from joining a religious cult.

The first time my doorbell rang, we were new to the neighborhood and I assumed the woman on my front stoop was my neighbor from across our backyard, out on an evening walk. I'm terrible with names and not so great with faces, so when she introduced herself and invited herself in, I assumed her name had just disappeared into the ether, along with the names and faces of most of my friends and family.

But then she started asking me about God, and what I thought happened after we died, and I realized this might not actually just be a neighbor rolling out the Welcome Wagon. The more I looked at her, I realized she wasn't the carefree softball mom who had introduced herself over my garden wall in the backyard. This lady had longer hair, puffier bangs. She was wearing a longer dress. A dress with very long sleeves. She had a pile of booklets with her. I had seen these booklets before, in New York, when women who looked like her wandered through the F train passing out "literature" about all the ways you may end up in hell, which read like a comic book about my twenties.

Very slowly, I realized she wasn't my neighbor. She didn't want to stop by for a glass of water. She wanted me to join her cult.

I remembered, suddenly, that I had to pick my child up from day care even though it was a Saturday afternoon. I promised this stranger that I would read her brochures and I thanked her for her concern over my mortal soul as I locked the door after her.

Never again, I thought, *never again.*

She returned a few months later. She'd spotted me through the picture window as she walked up to our house, and I answered the door because not hurting the feelings of a cult recruiter was more important to me than actually enjoying my afternoon. My mind was thinking, *Lady, could you please leave me alone? I am not interested in joining your cult.* But my stupid mouth was saying, "Nice to see you! Would you like a cup of coffee?" We talked a little bit about the brochures she had left, but mostly just about life and being moms. After an hour, I realized that I had a cult recruiter curled up on my couch and that she was playing the long con, and again, I used my son as an excuse so I wouldn't hurt her feelings and have her gossiping to God about me.

Month after month she returned for coffee and casual conversation. Sometimes, I would try just casually to mention that I was not in the market for a new religion. "Oh," I'd say, "my husband and I just went to a great meditation course. It was so open and accepting of different viewpoints." Or, "Our son was baptized at the Basilica in my old baptismal gown, isn't that neat?" She'd nod and smile and leave some more brochures on my coffee table. When I wasn't home, she'd leave a Post-it on my door or tell my baby-sitter to let me know she had stopped by.

When she left me her cell phone number, I knew things had gone too far, that I'd let the wrong one in and I was in danger of being eaten alive by a vampire.

So I made it stop. Finally. Because I stood up for myself and did what I should have done right away, the first time she showed up trying to sell me a new religion the way people sell knives or magazine subscriptions.

I moved.

Chapter 39

Meanwhile, the World Goes On

—MARY OLIVER

I cancelled my first date with Aaron to attend a funeral.

I don't even know if it would count as a date, but we were supposed to attend an advertising awards event together. It would most certainly have involved my getting far too drunk, far too fast, and him pouring me into his tiny VW Golf, dropping me on the curb outside of my apartment, and never speaking to me again. It's that kind of event. And I was that kind of girl.

Instead, I drove across the river to St. Paul in a black dress and met my mother in an elegant museum lobby. It was my first evening funeral, and it was . . . chic and beautiful, with passed hors d'oeuvres and theater seating. My mother and I took a seat near the aisle, and squeezed each other's hands three times.

Marshall died of glioblastoma, a brain tumor that crawled out from the center of his brain, snipping the wires that made him Marshall before destroying him completely.

His widow, Mary, went to grade school with my mother. At the funeral, Mary and her children were calm and peaceful in the face of a loss so big I could not comprehend it. Dads aren't supposed to die until their children are also old, when Dad is so old that you say, "Grandpa died," and your also-adult children can agree that it's for the best and say he had a good life and wonder aloud who is going to get his watches.

Dad is most definitely not supposed to die before his children are even all through high school. That is simply unacceptable.

You are sad for many reasons at a funeral. You are sad for the person who has died, for all of the people who loved that person. And you are sad for you, and the fact that you have loved people who are no longer here, people whose ghosts decide to sit with you through the service. And you're sad for our weak little mortal bodies and the fact that someday we will just be atoms floating through space and nobody will even remember our best tweets.

I cried for each of these reasons, all of them added up, like I had been storing up my sadness and cashed it all in at once. I have always wanted to be the kind of woman who was prepared for anything, who had a handbag with tissues on hand for moments like this, but I am not that kind of woman and all that was in my handbag were loose receipts and lip glosses and credit cards so instead I just wiped my nose on my sleeve.

MY MOTHER STAYED IN BED for weeks when her father died.

That can't actually be right, but that is how I remember that part of my childhood. The day our grandfather died, my little brother, Patrick, and I had had a very exciting afternoon with our own father. Outings with Steve were not regular occurrences. Dad worked a lot, even in the nineties before smartphones and email made it necessary for you to be tethered to your advertising job at all hours. Steve spent his free time golfing, a good game for a contemplative introvert with marginal athletic skills and a house full of noisy children. Our daily lives were attended to by our mother, who also worked a full-time job in advertising, but somehow managed to pack our lunches, sign our report cards, and remember to pick us up from school functions 40 percent of the time.

The time our dad spent with us was always generous and intoxicating. That day, he took us to see *The Three Musketeers* at the nearby movie theater, an old-fashioned joint with plush red seats and popcorn covered in real butter. As usual, he sat between us and ate all the best, most butter-soaked pieces before we even had a chance, but he'd bought us each our own "ice-cold Coca-Cola Classic," which is exactly how he insisted on ordering it at the counter, and a pack of Twizzlers to share. Afterward, we went to a local malt shop and washed our cheeseburgers down with a milk shake. I knew even in the moment that we were making a memory.

At home after the movie, my brother and I were high on life and refined sugar, reenacting scenes from the movie even though I was ten and right at the cusp of being too cool for that kind of thing. Patrick and I were engaged in a pretend sword fight, standing on his little twin bed wielding our paper towel tubes, when my father walked in and asked us to hold his hands and pray.

"Your grandfather just died," he said, the same way you might tell a child that dinner will be ready in twenty minutes. Patrick and I sat down on either side of our dad and held his hands the way we did nearly every Sunday at mass.

"Our Father, who art in heaven . . ."

Patrick, always so tender and open, wept against my father's shoulder until the prayer was done and Steve kissed us both and told us to be good, that our mother was going to need us. When our father left the room, Patrick turned to me, still sobbing, and I hugged him for as long as I could stand it while a tennis ball lodged in my throat.

My grandfather had not been sick. He had been old, I suppose, but only in the way that all grandparents are old—they are simply born at age seventy-five and remain there until you are old enough to understand how age works. Certainly there were older people on earth. My father had explained, briefly, how he had died: not of old age, but of a stroke, or something with his heart. I had tried to listen, but my mind was too busy serving me snapshots of my grandfather: his legs, spindly as a crane's from a childhood bout with rickets, wading after us into the cold of Lake Roosevelt; his thick Irish cable-knit sweater; the ceramic pot my grandmother had thrown for him in her studio, in which he hid his Brach's caramels, a treat he would sneak to us if we were good. The last time I had seen him was summer, up at the cabin where he lived with my grandmother, three hours from the city at the end of a dirt road. "You get more beautiful every day," he said to me when I got out of the car with a mouth full of crooked teeth and a boy's haircut.

Before I shut myself in my own bedroom, I snuck a peek down the hall toward the door of my parents' room. The afternoon light reduced everything in their room to its silhouette. There was the armoire, the big iron bed my parents shared, and the outline of my mother, under the covers, her back to the door. I could tell she was crying.

During that time, I don't remember my mother as anything but that silhouette. My father helped me pick out what to wear for the funeral. *The Addams Family* movie had recently come out, and I was hoping to wear something similar to Wednesday Addams's signature look, but they didn't have anything like that at Gap Kids, so I opted instead for a denim shirtdress with a black velvet collar. It didn't seem appropriate, but my dad told me that "children wearing black to a funeral is bullshit" so I accepted the dress and added a black beret to somber it up a bit.

I was annoyed a little with my mother, lying in bed while our father made us yet another plate of goddamn poached eggs and toast for dinner. Didn't she care that we had just lost our grandfather, for Pete's sake?

She must have been there, but I can't conjure her presence during that time, even at my grandfather's funeral. I had held my father's hand through the service, the skin tan and dry like fine-grit sandpaper, gripping mine like a vise during the Our Father.

I don't know when she came back to our world, just that one day she was there again, as if nothing had happened at all.

MY MOTHER LOOKS BEAUTIFUL AT my father's funeral. She is lean and elegant from years of yoga and a recent foray into the world of powerlifting. She has actually been in the local newspaper, in a feature on strength training and women, described as "a grandmother who can deadlift 135 pounds." Her record for deadlifts is actually 160 pounds, but we did not ask for a correction. Looking at her, with her cream-colored skin and her sky-blue eyes, her classic Diane Keaton style, I am reminded of the time my father told my high school boyfriend not to settle down with anyone (um, okay) until he'd taken a good look at her mother.

"Don't get too hung up on what she looks like now. If she's got a fat mom, there's no way around it, buddy, she's gonna get fat," he said.

"Now, you know Mary," he said of my grandmother, "I met her

when she was at least fifty, but she looked good. She still does. She doesn't look a day over eighty right now, which at her age is a big compliment."

My boyfriend at the time had nodded in agreement about the raw sexuality of my grandmother. He was always a good sport.

Your father's post-funeral luncheon is the saddest meal you'll ever eat, wedged between your father's funeral and his burial. We have overwhelmed the church ladies, who were not planning on feeding so many people ham sandwiches on white rolls and sides of goopy potato salad served with an ice cream scoop. They had tried in vain to get the crowd, a mix of devout and fallen-away Catholics, total heathens and other Minneapolis ad folk, to say a prayer before the meal was served, withholding the food under layers of plastic wrap. Finally, my cousin Johanna, a floaty, free, Northern California spirit, got one of them to give up control of the microphone, into which she had shouted, "Hey! Time to eat!" in place of the Lord's Prayer. "Ladies," she cooed to them as she returned the mic to its stand, "it's a funeral . . . relax." They have not relaxed, though, and they serve up the luncheon with a side of passive aggression. I sense that it is the wrong time to ask these women if there are any gluten-free options, so instead I drink cup after cup of strong black coffee in a laughably small disposable cup. In my big hands, it looks more like a thimble.

Aaron is sitting at a big round table with a group of my childhood friends, pushing food around his plate. He is wearing the suit my father helped him buy for our wedding, the one that cost more than twice my off-the-digital-rack wedding dress. It took both of us to get him into it today, as his growing brain tumor snips away at all of the functions we take for granted. He's a good sport as I button his shirt and buckle his belt and work his arm into a soft black sling I bought at the pharmacy. My dress does not have pockets, so Aaron has placed both my lipstick and my phone into the small pocket in his sling. "I'm just here to look good and be your living purse," he had said that morning as I adjusted his tie in the back of the church.

I've spent several hours pretending to know who I am talking to when they hug me and tell me how sorry they are for my loss, but most of these faces have meshed into one. Finally, there is one I know for certain, an old family friend who I am shocked to find has actually turned into an *old* family friend. He is handsome still, and older in the way they age movie actors in films where they need to play themselves in the future: like someone just drew some wrinkles on him with makeup and brushed some gray into his hair.

"Gosh," he says, looking past my shoulder to cast a loving, wistful gaze at my mother, "I always had such a crush on your mother."

After we bury my father, in a small plot among rolling acres of long-gone veterans, men and women whose lives are represented by identical white headstones, I go back to work. Everything at my little beige cube is exactly as I left it when I'd gotten a call from my sister the day before my father died telling me to leave work, now. My favorite mug is filled with a scummy layer of dried-up coffee, the highlighter I'd left uncapped is now dry. I spend the day staring blankly at my computer screen, getting hugs from coworkers who are very sorry to hear about my father, sitting in meetings and wondering how all of these people can carry on like this when there is such an obvious, gaping hole in the world. For days and weeks afterward, I pretend he is still alive, that he has left to spend the winter in Palm Springs as he had for years. I keep his number in my favorites, just in case I need to call him.

ONE SUMMER IN MY LATE twenties, I went to a funeral with my father for a person who was too young to die. It was early evening when the service ended, and when we made our way from the stony sadness of the viewing room to the outdoors, we found ourselves on a busy street with cars passing and late-summer sun shining and packs of young people, drunk on the feeling of being alive in the summer (and also beer), rushing down the sidewalk off to somewhere.

"That's the thing," my father said to me, my arm looped in his, "the world just keeps spinning, doesn't it?"

Chapter 40

Is He Going to Die Soon?

When your boyfriend is having his head shaved before emergency surgery to remove a brain tumor, the right thing to say about his shiny new head is probably not "You were going bald anyway." But that's what I said, because I am an idiot and because nobody ever knows what to say in awkward, terrible situations.

Aaron laughed, because he had the superhuman ability to laugh at himself, but even today I feel terrible about how that came out. Even though, I mean, I was right.

Since that bizarre *Twilight Zone* episode of a Halloween night where my boyfriend went from being a normal thirty-two-year-old dude to being a cancer patient, our family has gotten emails from long-lost acquaintances and friends of friends of friends. We have been stopped in restaurants and on the street by total strangers, people who just want to tell us they love our love, that they think of us often and wish us well. Even though this tends to happen when I am out in public wearing no makeup and looking like a drowned sewer rat, that's a really amazing feeling. It's been like a never-ending fire hose of love and energy that we get to dance in like sweaty children on a hot summer day, with occasional pauses for someone to instead pelt me in the face with a water balloon.

I feel like cancer is just a rite of passage, you know?
Yes! Cancer is just like getting hazed at your sorority or failing your driver's test because self-parking cars didn't exist in the nineties. I think you're on to something here.

So, is he going to die soon?
You know what? Great question. It's definitely not what a bride traditionally hears after her wedding, but that's what makes this such a memorable choice. Well done, former coworker.

My friend's husband had the EXACT SAME CANCER. He died.
Oh! Great! Please consider adding a spoiler alert to this conversation.

Have you tried a juice cleanse? Have you heard of Jim the Healer? He's located in Argentina, where he had to flee because the FDA didn't want him to cure cancer. He only takes American Express or PayPal. Here's the Geocities website he made in 1998.
Thank you so much for sharing your medical expertise. I know most people prefer to consult "doctors" about their cancer treatment, but why would we when you've got the answers?!

Do you think he would have married you if he didn't have cancer?

Well, there's only one way to tell: acquire a time machine, travel back in time and have him get a CAT scan in about 2006, when his brain tumor was probably just starting to form and was likely not yet cancerous. Then, conduct an elaborate scheme to get him to break up with his girlfriend and fall in love with me, and see if we still end up married. I'm guessing that tipping him off to the murderous cells hiding in his brain might help convince him to love me or totally freak him out, but it's worth a try!

You just have to keep fighting.

Yeah? I mean, cancer isn't much of a fight for some people. There are some where treatment is basically you just standing there while the Mike Tyson of cancers sucker-punches you over and over again. This is hard stuff, and a person can only take so much. When it's clear that it's time to call it, that's okay, too.

Don't worry, you're young. You'll find someone else.

Thank you for the pep talk. It's a really nice thing to hear at my husband's funeral. Do you think there's anyone here who is interested in dating me? Do you mind putting some feelers out for me?

I know how you feel. My [grandmother, dog, bus driver] just died and I am devastated.

Oh thanks yep you nailed it. You'll definitely feel the exact same way when your husband and father die right after your miscarriage.

You know, it's all a part of God's plan

Hey, God! Great plan! I *love* it. Super fun.

He's in a better place.
Like Martha's Vineyard?

It can be hard to know what to say to a person who is going through something difficult, but you can probably wipe these options from your list of conversation starters. There are no right words, though I wish there were because I would say them instead of the stupid, awkward shit that comes out of my mouth. If there were right words, I wouldn't have told my hysterical coworker to put her cat to sleep because it sounded like cat chemotherapy was kind of expensive.

You're thankful for the kind things people say, you forgive the dumb things, but you're crushed by the silence. I always like to think the best of myself, so I'd like to think that if something terrible happened to someone I knew, I'd be able to acknowledge it with love and encouragement, though I know it's easier said than done. When Aaron died, I heard from strangers around the world, but some of his closest friends disappeared completely. New friends came into my life, but some people I'd known forever didn't return.

I ran into my very first boyfriend the way Catholics tend to do . . . at a funeral. "I'm sorry," he said to me as he stood up from our lunch table in the church basement to head back to the office. "I never said anything to you about your dad or your husband. I didn't know what to say." We'd dated for nearly eight years, and my father had loved him and threatened to murder him on occasion. I'd noticed his absence in the piles of cards and emails I got after Aaron and my father died, and I let it burn me a little bit, to take the edge off the grief.

"I know," I told him, my heart cracking open just enough to feel for him, the mushroom-haircutted boy who'd kissed me on my parents' steps and always struggled to put his heart into words. I meant it—that I knew he didn't know what to say, and that I knew why.

"Nobody knows what to say. I don't even know what to say."

I don't worry so much about saying the right thing or the wrong thing anymore, and even all of the stupid things that people have said have a special place in my heart, because they're a sign that somebody tried. Sure, it was awkward and I wanted to punch a few throats, but being a human is awkward and uncomfortable. We're all just doing our best here. I have to remind myself of that all the time, especially since my Facebook feed has become 90 percent pyramid schemes involving either vitamins, essential oils, or nail decals.

Being a founder of the Hot Young Widows Club didn't bring me the wisdom to know what to say when I'm faced with death and sickness and grief. Most people are illiterate in the language of grief, and I count myself among that number. I am trying to learn and teach at the same time, but I am beginning to think that there is no right thing to say, and that perhaps it is okay for language to fail us at this time. It's okay for us to stumble for words when we're faced with death and sickness and grief; it's okay for stupid and awkward ones to slip out where we'd hoped sweet and comforting ones would have appeared.

You may be the person who says the wrong thing, but that's better than being the one who says nothing at all.

Chapter 41

"The Boy Is Mine"

I would really like to say that after I befriended my ex-boyfriend's new girlfriend and turned her into my lifelong friend I was forever cured of jealousy. And I do like to lie sometimes, but I still can't say that. I only lie about things like where I ate for lunch and why I couldn't make it to your birthday dinner. I don't lie about who I am because guess what? You're going to find out the truth eventually, when I die and I have nobody to clear my Google history for me.

On our second date, Aaron and I performed that delicate dance where you try to figure out just how available the person you're on a date with really is. You want to give out just enough information to let your paramour know that you've got no baggage and are footloose and fancy free, but not enough information that he knows you broke up with your last boyfriend via email because you're emotionally stunted. I went first, and tried to make it seem like I was ready for a boyfriend, but not *desperate* for one. When he asked if I was still friends with my exes, I changed the subject, as not a single one of them is currently on speaking terms with me. Maybe because I broke up with them via email or while riding bicycles? I wouldn't know, we don't speak anymore.

Aaron and his girlfriend had broken up pretty recently, he told me. Like, about a day before he and I met. Oh, and they'd dated for about a decade. Of course I couldn't be cool about this. He'd had *one* girlfriend and he dated her for nearly a third of his life.

It was clear to me that we couldn't date very seriously. I mean, I'd been through enough to realize that you don't build a successful relationship right on the heels of a failed one. You need to have a buffer of a few casual dates in between, a sort of sexual palate cleanser to get you ready for the next commitment.

In the few weeks that we'd known each other, we'd spent all day trading texts and Gchats and tweets, a constant stream of communication that I'd grown really fond of. Aaron was the first thing I saw in the morning, and the last thing I saw at night. Through my phone, but still. I was already attached. It had all been so devoid of the drama that underscored all of my previous romances. But then I had to find out that he'd had a girlfriend before me, and I felt that little green fire light up in my stomach again.

That night, at home in my apartment, I snapped in my retainer, opened my laptop, and prepared for my new case. I was back in the Facebook Forensics game, and I had a new mark.

It was easier than I thought. Aaron had a variety of Facebook albums for me to choose from, and they were rich with photos of a petite blonde, smiling and drunk and hanging all over him. She had long hair, a big smile, and a nose like mine. *So*, I thought, *he has a type.* I was able to put together a profile of my competition pretty quickly: His ex was named Nicole. She was shorter than me, which meant inferior. She was also a recent college graduate, and worked as a scientist. I wasn't wild about her being smarter than me, but reasoned that I probably made more money than her since I was more established in my career. Plus, Aaron and I both worked in advertising, so we'd have more to talk about, right? She seemed to be friends with all his friends, which was clearly going to be a problem, but they would probably grow to like me more once they got to know me. She may not be my next Karen, but we could probably be friends.

I was satisfied with my work, even if it took me a few weeks to realize that I was totally off and Nicole was Aaron's friend's little sister and not his former girlfriend.

So I started over. I had to dig deep this time, but I found her. His real ex. And the results did not look good for me. For one, she was taller than me. My résumé clearly states under "special skills" that I'm the tallest woman in the room, so I didn't like that development at all. She was also terribly pretty, like Mandy Moore only taller, an unfortunate combination for a fan of Mandy. She played college volleyball, unlike this quitter who stopped after high school. She had bigger boobs than me for sure, though there are ten-year-olds who have achieved the same thing. To top it off, she was barely even on the Internet. It was like she had a rich, satisfying life offline or something. I wasn't pleased.

Unlike me, who would tell you literally anything you wanted to know about any guy I've ever so much as kissed, Aaron was really respectful about his relationship with Katie. It just wasn't meant to be, he'd say, and then that would be that, and I would just be left to wonder if she wore makeup or if her skin was really that good.

Even though in my heart I knew that if I could just *Parent Trap* us together I could win her over the way I'd won over Karen and we could be best friends who got manicures together and talked about Aaron's faults behind his back, I had no choice but to consider the case closed. Until that tall, beautiful dame walked back into my life.

We were in the pre-op room in the basement of the hospital about two minutes before doctors were going to chainsaw Aaron's head open to take out a brain tumor we'd just found out about. So, you could say that the atmosphere was a little intense. When the curtains opened, I expected it to be the little old nurse who had left abruptly when a drugged-up Aaron accused her of "trying to get up on my diiiiiick," but instead, it was Katie.

It was immediately clear that she had as good an idea as I did as to how she'd ended up back here, and my hard little Grinch heart softened into a little sponge. I wanted to hug her, but there wasn't enough room, so I just extended my arm and we shook hands over Aaron's half-conscious body. Per my "meeting girls I've stalked" code, I hadn't showered in many days, and had my hair in a greasy bun. She did look exactly like a taller Mandy Moore. And she smelled nice. And then, she was gone.

While Aaron's surgery got under way, I walked through the cold, sterile halls of the hospital until I got to the adjoining hotel, where I took the kind of long, hot shower that burns off at least a layer of skin and helps you think all of the thoughts you've been too tired to think. I realized, standing in a Marriott shower while my boyfriend had what the doctors referred to as a "skull flap" cut into his cranium, that love was the best thing to have in common with anyone. It was a goddamn Carrie Bradshaw moment. I loved Aaron, and so had Katie. So I loved Katie, too. For spending her adolescence with the man I would marry, and for setting him free just in time.

I didn't see her again for years, even though we became Facebook friends and exchanged phone numbers and liked each other's Instagram photos and I referred to her as "my friend Katie" like we had in fact gone to school together and not just loved the same dude at different times. I spotted Katie while I delivered Aaron's eulogy, her pretty face floating head and shoulders above the crowd. And after hugging about seven hundred people and slamming as many glasses of white wine, I cornered her, held her in my sweaty arms, and begged her to come out to the bar with us afterward. And, like a best friend I had only met once before, she did.

It was the karaoke bar where she and Aaron had spent many nights, and Aaron and I had gone when we started dating. I put in my request right away. A duet that I normally performed myself, though tonight I was ready to share the stage. What video footage from that night tells me is that when we took the stage, we crushed it. And by crushed it I mean it is not clear that I am singing the right song, and somebody unplugged my microphone without me even noticing. But I don't remember any of that, so who cares.

I just remember Katie smiling at me, holding my sweaty hand, and agreeing to sing with me. "What song?" she asked me, walking up to the stage.

" 'The Boy Is Mine.' "

Chapter 42

Welcome to Grey Gardens

This is a just a temporary roommate situation. It's not like I *live* with my mom—that would be crazy. Besides, we've tried that before a few times and it always ended up with one of us (her) recommending the other one (me) get an apartment. I told her the last time she kicked me out that this was it, I wasn't going to be returning to the nest just to eat her food and not pay rent, and if she thought I was going to, she had another thing coming. At the time, she and my father had some annoying habits they weren't ready to confront, like grinding coffee at 7:00 A.M. even when I had a hangover, or always wanting to know when I was coming back just because I was driving their car.

That was when I was young, just a tender little angel at the age of twenty-seven, smoking cigarettes on the back steps and spraying myself with Febreze to hide the smell. Now I'm an adult woman with a child and a 401(k), I don't *live* with my mom. I don't sleep in the bed I got when I was sixteen and finally convinced my parents that I was too tall for a twin with a footboard, why would you even think that? Yes, I woke up there this morning but it was more like I just needed a place to crash, and I was already at my mom's house and had already put my son to bed in the room next door, and my toothbrush was already here, so I figured, hey, why not take a snooze? Yes, my son and I have been spending seven nights a week at my mom's place for the past few months but it's not like we *live* there. It's not like she buys our groceries or has accidentally worn my underwear. That's just gross, you weirdo.

Yes, I did get your letter but it took a while to get to me because my mail is being forwarded from our actual house—the one that we own—to my mom's place, just for safekeeping. And sometimes my mom puts my mail in these annoying little piles and I miss things like my bills or my proof-of-insurance cards.

Sure, we'd joked about it, before, how the two of us would end up together like Big and Little Edie, a house crumbling around us while we slowly lose our minds. But that doesn't mean we'd move in together just because we're both widows. And even if we did, what's next? You think we're going to get a hot plate and start cooking up corn by the side of our bed? Just because it's convenient and boiled corn on the cob is a seasonal treat, particularly in Minnesota, where our sweet corn just cannot be topped?

Without my father's fastidiousness and judgment to hold her down, my mother has a newfound freedom from things like cleaning or dusting or taking the laundry out of the wash and putting it in the dryer before it grows mildew. That's not entirely fair; I did see her scrubbing out a trash can with the same brush we use to wash the dishes, and she pointed out that "things like this" are why I have such a good immune system. And that is a solid point, but still, my son often picks up entire dust bunnies with his hands and declares the house "TOO DIRTY" but he's two, there's no making a two-year-old happy. Plus, he doesn't exactly pitch in, so it's not like he's really in the position to be throwing stones here. He didn't even thank us when we hung sheets over his windows because the room he's crashing in gets too bright in the morning. He just said something about us being hillbillies and hadn't we ever heard of room darkening shades?

The boxes you tripped over in the living room are the contents of my closet. You can tell because they're labeled NORA'S CLOTHES and there are hangers sticking out of them every which way. I'd hang my clothes up, but all of the closets are full, and besides, it doesn't bother me just to walk down here in the morning and rifle through a few piles of my things before selecting an outfit. It's basically just a storage unit, but right in the living room, so way easier than a storage unit, because I don't need to drive down to some frontage road off the highway and then pretend not to notice the people who are living in an eight-by-ten steel box filled with old doll parts. Instead, I can have all the benefits of a storage unit in the privacy of my mother's home.

We don't have any pets *yet* because cats poop in the house and dogs poop in the yard and right now, Ralph gives me more than enough poop to clean up. I'm hoping that he'll be potty trained soon but he seems to really enjoy the feeling of hot poop pressed up against his man parts. So, no pets yet but I will say that if either of us found a baby raccoon, yeah, we'd probably take it in. Have you seen their hands? They have people hands! How can you resist that? Are you dead inside? I have also been eyeing the albino squirrel that pops up in our neighborhood. I heard that they're lucky.

What am I *wearing*? I'm wearing a head wrap. It used to be a skirt. Thank you, I know, it *does* look good.

Yes, we do have Wi-Fi here. The network is called Grey Gardens. Welcome.

Chapter 43

Petty Crimes

aron wasn't afraid of dying of cancer. He was afraid of dying because I started a fight over something petty with a stranger, who then shot at me, but missed and killed Aaron. From our very first date, Aaron loved absolutely everything about me except for the smell of my armpits ("What are you eating that makes you smell like a garbage dump?"), my nose picking ("Where do you put the boogers?"), and my need to police our community for petty crimes ("Please don't wag your finger at that man for texting at a stoplight").

I think part of him was proud of my thirst for justice, because he always told me I could star in a crime show called *Petty Crimes*, where I'd play a version of myself named Nicole Petty, because people really love TV shows that pun on the names of the lead character. Nicole would be a really cool, smart, tall woman with smelly armpits who spent her free time as a volunteer police officer, an honor that has only been extended to Shaq and Steven Seagal. Nicole would spend her time taking care of the petty crimes, like people smoking next to NO SMOKING signs right outside of the oncology building at the hospital, or people who turn left on a red arrow, so the cops could round up the real bad guys. It would likely air late night. Like Dick Wolf, Aaron ripped from the headlines, and found his inspiration in the times I followed the teenagers who were snorting Adderall on our steps and talked to their high school principal about their drug habits or the time I left a note saying, "This is not nice," to the person who parked so close to our car that I had to climb in through the passenger side to drive.

My passion for the law and its obedience started young, when I was just a run-of-the-mill tattletale, snitching on everyone for everything. When you are one of four children, it's necessary to keep score, and you can't keep score without taking careful notes on any rule infractions by your competitors and reporting them to the necessary authorities. In grade school, we had to watch some sort of video once about how tattling was bad. In it, a rattlesnake sang about how when his tongue started to tattle, his tail started to rattle. And it was hard for me to understand, because that is just biologically incorrect and also because why was it bad for me to point out how other people were being bad? Shouldn't the teacher be concerned that Sean Johnson put Jordan Peterson's jacket in the toilet and peed on it? Shouldn't my mother know that my little brother wasn't just "going for a walk" with his friends, they were "going for a walk in order to smoke pot"? Aren't those important facts?

An important thing happened to me in high school, and that thing was a class called Street Law. It was taught by one of our history teachers, and it was the most sought-after class you could take. In it, we learned all kinds of ways to be street smart, like what our rights were if the cops stopped our car, and when and how to perform a citizen's arrest. Most of the curriculum was taught through reruns of *Law & Order,* and from the first time I heard the *dun-dun* of the opening credits, I was hooked. Here was an entire show based around people finding other people doing wrong things, documenting their offenses, and being rewarded for their efforts instead of being told, "Nora, please stop talking and go back to your desk." I'd found the passion that would sustain me for the rest of my life. That year, I also took my first trip to New York City, where my father gave me $50 to spend however I wanted and I gave it all to a homeless man outside the Times Square Hilton because he said he didn't have any money at all. I also met Richard Belzer, aka Munch from *Law & Order: SVU.* He seemed shocked to be recognized by two teenage girls, and extremely uncomfortable when we started to cry. "We watch your show in school!" we told him as he reluctantly signed an autograph using a CoverGirl eyeliner I'd fished out of my backpack. "That's really not appropriate," he replied.

But Munch was wrong. Watching *Law & Order: SVU* was very appropriate and very awesome, and I learned a lot about what can happen on a New York City rooftop if you're not careful. I also realized that I could have an entire career based on being a snitch and a tattletale, and I looked forward to my career as a sexy prosecutor, sexy detective, or sexy forensics expert. I embraced my purpose in life with a new kind of zeal. I rolled down my window at stoplights to tell people that their blinkers or brake lights weren't working, and it was time to get their old jalopy to the shop right away. I got a job as a lifeguard and banned three different adult males old enough to be my father for diving in shallow water. When they protested and threatened to call the city to complain about me, I stood proudly in my red suit and Ray-Bans and told them to go ahead and call, because I was right and they were wrong. Rules were rules, and they were clearly posted at the pool entrance.

I was a pretty chill teenager.

One sunny fall morning, driving my mother's lime green VW Beetle to my senior year of high school, I saw another offense that needed correcting. A family van with clearly only one passenger was sailing onto the freeway just ahead of me, illegally using the carpool lane to avoid the metered entrance.

But not on my watch.

I laid on the horn while my best friends Erica and Barb booed along with me. They weren't natural crime fighters, but they at least appreciated my enthusiasm for justice. We held up our middle fingers as the silhouette of the driver in front of us held up his hands in surrender.

"Hands on the wheel, buddy!" I yelled, honking again.

Usually, cars with grown-ups in them would peel off 35 North directly into the heart of downtown. But this van didn't do that. Instead, we followed it past the downtown exits, toward the University of Minnesota, where we exited to follow the Mississippi right onto Nicollet Island. And into our high school parking lot. Where our principal got out of the car, looked at us, and slid open the door of his family van, to let out his youngest daughter.

I got all the way to lunch period without seeing him, but there he was. Had he waited for me in the lunchroom? And could he legally expel me in public? With all these witnesses?

"Nora!" he said, in his big, friendly voice. It was hard not to love this jolly perp, but I tried to stay stern.

"I think I saw you getting on the freeway this morning, in the carpool lane?" He was getting nervous now, so maybe I wasn't expelled?

"I just wanted you to know that I know you think I cheated, but I didn't. I know it doesn't seem right, but a two-year-old does make it a valid carpool."

I nodded and considered his testimony.

"You're right, it really doesn't seem right to me. But don't worry, sir. We're cool." I walked to my lunch table feeling small and guilty for making a grown adult male feel he had to explain himself to me for a crime he didn't even commit.

The day after Aaron's funeral, I woke up with that same sick little feeling in my heart, the sense that I'd gone a little too far. I also woke up with a sick feeling in my head, stomach, arms, fingernails, and hair because I was in the midst of the worst hangover of my entire life, one where the previous night was just a blur of images that my brain could not bring into focus.

Blacking out when you're drinking is never a great thing to do, but I would say that it's not a particularly becoming thing to do directly after your husband's funeral. I remember the parts I was sober for, like the funeral itself, but the after-party was drenched in whiskey and karaoke. Oh, karaoke! Did I sing both sides of the Meat Loaf hit "Anything for Love"? Yes, yes, I did. A few scenes come back to me. I felt like I sounded somewhere between great and awesome, but I also vaguely recall an entire bar filled with people staring at me in jaw-dropping horror.

And then I remember. Aaron's friend Bryce. A groomsman in our wedding three years before, to the day. Whom we hadn't really seen since. Who hadn't come to meet our son, now two, though Aaron waited up for him the night after chemo, when Bryce had promised to stop by. He was one of many friends, actually, who hadn't shown up for us, who hadn't wanted to face Aaron's death or sickness, and had left us to deal with it alone. But he was also the only one who had the guts to try to apologize to me when I was blackout drunk at my husband's funeral.

It was . . . not the right time.

Which I let him know. I let him know everything I had been

feeling for the past three years, and then some. I was ruthless and biting, and I remember our friends pulling him away from me, tears rolling down his face while I all but licked his blood from my claws and slammed another whiskey-ginger.

Bryce had the same reasons for not being there that everyone who wasn't there had: they didn't want to ruin their memories of him, they didn't want to be sad, they were scared, they didn't know what to do.

Nicole Petty would not stand for that. Because Aaron didn't want to do any of this, either, but he didn't have a choice. You don't get to just come to the wedding and the funeral, but skip the middle part because it might make you too sad. *That is against the rules.*

It took me months to realize I was wrong, because I didn't have Aaron to tell me what he'd told me when I'd been sharp and defensive on his behalf, when people who were supposed to be close to him failed to be there for him. Not everyone does what they're supposed to do, or does what you want them to do. And sure, it can hurt your feelings, or annoy you, but it's not a crime. We are people and we do lots of things we can't explain, like go to Donald Trump rallies or believe that Apple is giving away "broken" iPads through comments on a Facebook post. We're just humans, and humans are weird and scared and dumb. We fuck up. But that doesn't make it a crime.

It's not up to Nicole Petty to exact justice for every infraction; there are bigger problems in the world, like people who don't properly signal their turns, or who litter out their car window on the freeway.

Bryce forgave me, even though he didn't have to, because he's clearly a better person than I am. Nicole Petty retired her badge. Unless you're texting and driving, in which case, look out. The long arm of the law is coming for you.

Chapter 44

Lean In

The bar is really low when it comes to fatherhood. I realized this when nurses were excited that Aaron was going to be in the delivery room, like a guy who has put his penis in my vagina should be nervous about seeing what comes out of it. But it just got worse. If Aaron held Ralph or engaged with him in any way in public, strangers would shower him with approval.

"What a *great* dad!" waiters would say when Aaron handed Ralph his sippy cup.

"What a *great* dad!" strangers at the mall would say if Aaron was holding him.

"What a *great* dad!" old ladies would coo if Aaron pushed the stroller in the park.

When Ralph was nearly a year old, he and Aaron took a standby flight to Atlanta to visit Aaron's sister and her family. They waited an entire day for two seats to open up, and Aaron and Ralph spent the entire flight being doted on by attendants who were so charmed by the idea that a man and his child could fly across the country without female supervision. Meanwhile, I could be carrying a car seat, a giant diaper bag, and two shopping bags out of Target and people would honk at me to get out of their way in the parking lot or criticize me because they caught a little side boob while I was nursing Ralph on an airplane.

I don't say this to imply that Aaron wasn't a great dad; he was an awesome dad for the year and a half he got to be one, but not because he did the bare minimum of parenting.

Ralph was born when Aaron was starting a gnarly version of chemo that meant he would be hospitalized for at least three days every month, while the doctors snaked a needle through the artery in his leg, all the way up to his brain, where they would squirt in poison and hope it killed the tumor instead of Aaron.

It was risky and painful, and it left him feeling like shit.

But you'd never know it.

Right after Ralph was born, I got a double ear infection. You would have thought that I was the one diagnosed with a terminal brain tumor, because I laid in bed crying and cursing the world, and then broke out in a full-body rash because it turned out I was also allergic to antibiotics. Meanwhile, Aaron changed Ralph's tiny diapers, refilled the small squirt bottle of water I needed to keep by the toilet to flush out the stitches holding my vagina together, and watched every episode of *Girls* even though he was uncomfortable with how much I related to the show.

While I was on maternity leave, he special-ordered the book *Lean In* and left it on my bedside table. I read it at night while I was nursing Ralph and Aaron was reading his comic books, and I had to stop every few lines to read something out loud to him, because when Sheryl Sandberg wrote about having a true partner, she was writing about both our husbands.

I was ready when I went back to work, but my brain was not,

and I found even basic tasks of adulthood completely slipping my mind. Things like turning off the burners when I was done using them, or remembering to pack a diaper for Ralph when we left the house.

Every day, I got close to the end of my rapidly fraying rope, and Aaron would give me a boost so I could climb back up. "Leave me a list of what you want done tomorrow," he'd say, and if I didn't do it, he'd text me all day asking for things to take off my plate.

The first six months of a baby's life are supposed to be massively stressful, probably more so when your husband is also undergoing treatment for a disease that will eventually kill him. But it felt light and easy most days, because Aaron was there so fully. "Do you want to go to yoga tonight?" he'd ask me in the morning. "I can put Ralphie to bed."

But instead of going to bed on time, they'd stay up goofing around and listening to records, and when I snuck in the back door to keep from waking the baby, I'd hear Aaron singing "Thunder Road" to Ralph in the rocking chair. When he could no longer be alone with Ralph, or lift him on his own, he'd still find his ways to lean in. He'd call friends to come over and hang out with him and help put Ralph to bed so I could go to the gym; he'd order our groceries online and make sure we had tickets to every good concert in Minneapolis.

He was a really good father, a really good husband, and a damn good partner, two other categories in which the bar is often lowered so far that men are in danger of tripping over it. He was a great partner not in spite of his cancer, or because of it, but completely apart from it, because he didn't want to let it affect his contribution to our relationship in any way.

One Sunday afternoon, I found myself in the living room of a former coworker who talks to dead people. It's a skill she was born with, being able to relay messages between two worlds, like a living answering machine. If this sounds nuts to you, you'd just have to meet this tall, willowy human with her wild mane of black hair and her unfailing eye contact, and you'd totally believe. And it sounded a little nuts to me, but Catholics believe that if we lose our car keys there's a specific saint who can help us find them, so is it really that outlandish to think that a former project manager of mine could help me speak with my dead husband?

There was nothing ceremonial about it, either. One moment, we were sitting in Cecilia's cozy living room, my feet tucked under me on her sofa, a plate of cookies between us on her antique coffee table, gossiping about old coworkers. And then, she announced that Aaron was here, waving her arm to indicate that he was somewhere between the curio cabinet and the picture window. "Hi." I waved to the empty room between us, suddenly shy and self-conscious.

"He says hi, but he's not saying Nora. He's saying something else. Norn?"

"Yeah?" I know that it really is Aaron. When I met him, I told him Nora was a hard name to nickname as a kid. He didn't miss a beat. "Nobody called you Chronicles of Nornia?" he asked, and that was my name, until he shortened it to Nornia. Or Norn.

I was a little shy at first, because it had been a while since I'd talked to Aaron, but nothing had really changed. We were still on the same team. He told me to move out of our house; it was too hard for me to be there and the home had served its purpose in our lives. It was time to go, as soon as I could.

He told me I was doing a good job, but that I needed to buck up a little and be the crazy bitch he'd fallen in love with, who stood up for herself and the people around her. I'd recently had some bizarre interpersonal experiences that the Nora he loved would have never stood for, and I nodded in agreement and let the tears I'd been blinking back fall into my lap.

It was nice to talk to him again, like no time had passed, like he hadn't died in my arms months before. Like we weren't communicating through a woman I hardly knew, who sat in her armchair, staring dreamily out the window while our tea went cold.

He wanted a to-do list.

A to-do list? What would I possibly ask him to do, pick Ralph up from day care?

"I can still help you," he told me, "just write it all down and I'll find someone who can do it."

And then he was gone, and Cecilia and I were just two former colleagues who had communed with the afterworld before lunch.

I pulled over a block from her house and dug through my purse for a notebook. *HELP ME, AARON,* I wrote on the top of the page, and made a list:

- I need Ralph to sleep through the night

- I need someone to rent our house

- Where will we live next?

- I need to be happier and more peaceful

- I need to love again. Not yet. But someday? Is that okay?

I dog-eared the page, started the car, and I went on with my life. And things started happening.

Ralph stopped waking up hysterical in the middle of the night, and the fog around me lifted. The first house I looked at with a realtor seemed perfect, and then I got to the kitchen. The fridge was free of the debris a normal family fridge is covered in: save-the-dates and finger paintings and free magnets from your local pizza shop. There was just one little piece of paper, the prayer card from Aaron's funeral, telling me, "It's Going to Be Okay."

After investigating the rest of the property, I found a wedding photo, and saw that the bride was a classmate from grade school.

"Hey," I messaged her through Facebook. "I'm in your house right now and your dog is licking my leg."

This was clearly meant to be, and Aaron had led me right to my destiny.

Even though she and her husband accepted an offer thirteen minutes after I toured their place, she got in touch when I listed my own house for rent and signed a lease immediately.

One by one, I checked things off the list I had made for Aaron, and added new ones, because I know that's what he would want.

Maybe it's all one big coincidence, and maybe you're all rolling your eyes at me right now. I don't care. I know that Aaron is dead. But I also know that he is still leaning in to this marriage.

It's time to raise the bar, fellas.

Chapter 45

Just Quit

There's a pivotal scene in MTV's *The Hills* that nobody but my best friend Dave and I remember, when Heidi Montag still looks like Heidi Montag and she's dating a guy named Jordan. Heidi has gotten a very coveted PR job in Los Angeles, but it comes with the unfortunate requirement that she go to the office and *work* every day, which doesn't really leave her a lot of time to hang out in bed with Jordan. One morning, while she's getting ready to start her day like a responsible young adult, Jordan urges her to instead dedicate herself to staying in bed all day.

"Quit," Jordan whispers in her ear.

But Heidi doesn't quit. She goes to work and orders sandwiches and books travel for her boss. Or, I mean, she is filmed doing that. Most of the Internet agrees that her job was fake but just stick with me here. If you don't know who Heidi Montag is, it's because this began her rapid demise. Instead of dethroning Lauren Conrad as the queen of Southern California reality TV and transitioning into a career as an Internet fashion mogul, she ended up as a cautionary tale married to a reality TV villain with blond facial hair who collects crystals.

All because she didn't follow Jordan's questionable advice, and quit.

If Aaron were alive, lying in bed next to me while I whined about what to do for the day, he would for sure be sexy-whispering R. Kelly songs because we thought it was hilarious to whisper them to each other.

Like Heidi, I don't want to go to work anymore. Not because I have a lazy boyfriend who just wants to have sex with me all day (I WISH), but because I just don't want to do anything at all. Grief is kind of a full-time job, and when you add in a toddler and the fact that *Gilmore Girls* is now on Netflix, I'm working double overtime right now. I don't have time to wake up, shower, eat breakfast, put on an outfit and go to *work,* where inevitably they will ask me to do things and go to meetings and answer questions. I know I'm supposed to do that, but after looking over my schedule, I just don't see work fitting in anywhere.

Something inside me, possibly that third glass of rosé, tells me it's time to quit my job and be a single, stay-at-home mother whose child is in day care full-time. That something is definitely not my financial planner, whose advice was *not* to quit my job, and instead *keep* my job, as having a steady source of income would be wise as a single woman. She has done a lot for our family, like explaining to me and Aaron that Nikes are not an actual investment, and that there are places to put our money that aren't our closets. Still, I think she may be wrong about this one.

I am not sure if quitting my job is going to signal my own Heidi Montag–level breakdown or help me avoid one, but I'm willing to risk it anyway. I mean, what's the worst that can happen? My husband and dad can't die again, and jobs are like bobby pins:

you can lose a thousand of them, but you always find another one. I'm just not interested in pretending that I still have the life I used to have, where I had a husband and a baby and a normal job. That life died when Aaron did, and I'm still trying to figure out what this new life looks like, like the girl I used to dance on the bar with in college who is now a Catholic nun.

Like most Midwesterners, I was raised to appreciate perseverance. Your marriage should last at least fifty years and end when one of you dies. When the going gets tough, the tough get going. So I did a lot of things I didn't want to do, just because they were expected of me. I played basketball just because I was tall, even though I spent most games after turning fourteen just sitting on the bench, avoiding eye contact with my coach and hoping I wouldn't have to sweat and ruin my makeup. I stayed with a boyfriend twice as long as I should have because when I was like "let's break up," he was like "no, thanks." I did that more than once, with boys and with jobs, because somewhere along the line I'd absorbed the idea that it's not good to have too many of either of those things. But why not? Dating a lot of boys and having a lot of jobs should tell you that I'm interested in finding the one that's right for me, not just hunkering down and suffering through sex with someone whose bones protrude so far I can actually hear our skeletons clanking together, or a job where my boss thinks that the pizza we are eating for lunch is topped with "shit-talking mushrooms." I refuse to let people slut-shame me for having a lot of jobs. I watched two different people die last year, and neither one of them was like "oh, gosh, if I have one regret it's based around my employment history."

The happiest people in my life are people who did the thing our coaches and parents always told us not to do: They quit. And once they do, they wonder what took them so long, and why they had been so dedicated to something they disliked so much. Before you're, like, okay, wow, what a privileged point of view, let me tell you, *yep*.

But I'm not just talking about job quitters, because yes, it's a privilege to have a safety net that lets you just quit your job to figure out who you are and that shit doesn't always work out for everyone because life is not an indie movie about finding yourself through a passion for artisanal soaps.

I'm just talking about not doing the things you hate doing anymore. Aside from paying your taxes and flossing, which are nonnegotiable. But most of what we don't want to do are not things we actually *have to do.*

When the pressures of digital relationships detract from real-life relationships, sign out. Give the password to your best friend and tell her to keep you out for a few weeks. When you go back, you'll have missed nothing but a few birthdays of people whose birthdays obviously weren't that important to you in the first place or they'd already be in your calendar. Trust me, if your sister has a baby, you'll find out even without Facebook. Then, you can go on an unfollowing spree, cleansing your feed of every person who still says "Bruce Jenner" or abuses Facebook in the name of "network marketing," which used to just be called a pyramid scheme.

You don't actually have to hang out with people who make you feel exhausted or take little digs at you. You know how everyone has a friend who is basically just mean to them, and you can't figure out why you are friends with this girl who says things like "Did you guys totally give up on trying to have nice things when you had a kid?" while she's sitting on a couch that you are proud to say has very few visible boogers crusted onto it? You don't need to go to her home-shopping party and buy a bunch of personalized bags you'll never use.

If you're married to a total butthole who doesn't keep up his end of the bargain? Quit. Marriage isn't supposed to feel like a cage, it's supposed to feel like a hug that lasts just a few seconds too long.

Now, is not quitting her job directly related to where Heidi ended up in life? For the sake of this essay, the answer is yes because she stayed at that job, broke up with Jordan, and ended up with Spencer and zero friends. What is not debatable is that some of our greatest treasures are ours because they were big old quitters. You think you'd see old people grinding to "SexyBack" at every single wedding if Justin were still in N*SYNC? I doubt it. Don't you appreciate *30 Rock* more knowing that it was possible because Tina Fey quit working at *Saturday Night Live*? Isn't it amazing that Robert Downey Jr., used to be a huge mess but then he quit drugs and now our kids can watch him save the world as Iron Man?

The world will keep spinning, and your life will get a little bit better every time you give up on the shit that is taking you away from your one wild and precious life. Nobody is making you go to coffee with that guy you haven't seen since middle school who is going to try to get you to buy a time-share; nobody is making you stay up until 2:00 A.M. making "end of school" gift bags for forty-eight seven-year-olds or accept Facebook invites to birthday dinners you'd rather not attend. These things aren't jobs, but they feel like them. So let me be your Jordan, whispering gently into your ear, only pushing you toward better things in life because I have your best interests at heart and I'm not sleeping with you.

Quit.

Chapter 46

It's Going to Be Okay
(I Think)

When your dying husband wants pancakes, you get him some fucking pancakes. If ever there is a time to eat your feelings, this would be it, but I cannot. In part because I do not have much of an appetite, and in part because my doctor recently informed me that I can no longer enjoy foods that contain gluten, or in other words, that I can no longer enjoy any of the foods that I consider foods. "Nora," Aaron said emphatically when I shared my diagnosis with him, "this might be the worst thing that ever happens to you."

The diner is small—just a few tables and some stools at the counter, so small that Aaron and I are actually too big to sit there, though before my gluten issues, we would do it just for the chance to eat these pancakes, bigger than our heads, sizzling on a griddle that's older than the two of us combined. The lunch rush is over, but a few wayward teens with Technicolor hair and safety pin earrings sit a few feet from us. Nobody, I realize, knows that Aaron is dying. It is our little secret. There are many reasons for people to explain why I am crying into my coffee. We could be getting a divorce or being evicted from our apartment or have an inkling that the $20,000 we sent to secure our million-dollar inheritance from a long-lost Nigerian uncle might not pan out.

Or maybe they do know that Aaron is eating the very last public meal of his life. It may not be as mysterious as I think it is. I'd taken the one handicapped parking spot, though our application was still finding its way through the bureaucracy of the DMV. There were already a few snowbanks, and to get Aaron from the car to the sidewalk, I'd had to squat down and lift him from the waist, like two figure skaters in a dry rehearsal. "Watch my nuts!" he'd yelled, resting his good arm on top of my head like this was a completely natural situation for any couple to be in.

"So," Aaron asks me as he hands me the butter knife to cut his pancakes, "what do you want to do now? Should we go to Italy? Should we go to Brazil?"

There will be no trip to Italy or Brazil, but we talk about it anyway, one last little kindness in a sweet little lie.

"I just want to be here," I say, "with you."

WE'D STARTED THAT DAY IN the same emergency room he'd been admitted to three years earlier. That first day, before brain cancer was even a part of our vocabulary, was like a field trip for us. We'd found it all so outrageous and fascinating: Why would they make Aaron stay in the hospital, just because he'd had a seizure? Didn't they know he was young and healthy? That we'd just moved in together, and weren't planning to tell my parents about the cohabitation? I was only just beginning to shake off the hangover from the Halloween party he'd thrown on Saturday night, so I was having a particularly hard time keeping up with even normal conversations, let alone whatever medical nonsense the nurses were spouting whenever they stepped into our little space in the emergency room. Aaron had given me his phone that afternoon and told me to Instagram everything. I took a handsome photo of him as a modern-day FDR: his skinny legs in the nonslip socks they insist you wear, poking out from under the blanket on his lap as we wheelchaired him to his MRI. We didn't really know what an MRI was, just that he needed to get one, so that we could get home and get on with our lives, which for me meant chugging at least fifty more ounces of Gatorade and eating a cheeseburger on our couch while Aaron handed out the Halloween candy. I sat on Aaron's lap in the wheelchair while we waited for his name to be called, his thumb tracing little infinity signs on the small of my back, the way he did every time we touched. Next to us, there was an old man lying alone on a hospital bed, motionless except for the rise and fall of his chest and the occasional blink of his watery eyes.

We assumed he was first in line.

When it was Aaron's turn, I followed him right to the door of the room where what looked like a small spaceship was waiting for him. It took a team of people in various shades of pastel scrubs to get him all strapped in, and before they shut the door I could hear him calling my name. A small part of me, the part that wasn't thinking of quippy tweets and flirting with Aaron in the basement of a hospital, knew that we were in a Moment. That there would be Before this moment and After, and I tried to take in everything that I could, to reassemble for future contemplation. Like, for example, how he called out for me before they shut the door.

"Nora," he called, raising his arm and gesturing with his forefinger as I stepped closer. "Take a picture for Instagram."

SINCE THEN WE'D BECOME ER professionals, prepared for a full day of bullshit: two laptops, two iPads, two iPhones, our own chargers for each device, a pile of fresh comic books for Aaron, San Pellegrino water, KIND bars, and Sour Patch Kids. Before the nurse has even pulled the curtain shut, I've pulled the folding chairs from their hanging spot on the wall and kicked off my shoes, putting my feet up on the foot of Aaron's hospital bed and blindly accepting the terms and conditions for the free hospital Wi-Fi, which probably means I've forfeited all rights to my internal organs in exchange for a snail's-pace crawl toward the information superhighway. There's no Instagram today—Aaron doesn't want his mother to worry about him (World's Best Son Award)—but we settle into our routine of finding funny tweets to read aloud to one another. I suck at this because I can't get through more than three words of anything Jenny Mollen writes without giggling like I'm in church and just heard somebody fart, but Aaron finds gem after gem, and we may as well be at home in bed except for the sound of a woman howling outside of our room, begging to be put into rehab, insisting she was ready to get clean. "That lady thinks she's done some shit?" Aaron sighed, staring at the ceiling. "She should try chemo. That's the really hard stuff."

The ER doctor is *Grey's Anatomy*–level hot, the kind of tall, corn-fed good looks you really only see in Midwestern men. I have my suspicions, at first, that he is just pretending to be a doctor, some sort of hired eye candy the hospital sends to particularly tense situations just to add a little sexiness to the atmosphere. He listens carefully while Aaron describes his last seizure, and orders up an emergency MRI, bumping Aaron to the top of the list.

"Is it just me . . . ," I say after Dr. McDreamy leaves the room.

"No, he's hot," Aaron interjects, "but cool your jets, I'm not dead yet."

This time, I don't follow Aaron in a wheelchair. They push him down there in his bed, just like that milky-eyed old man we'd seen three years ago. I wonder whatever became of that guy, though I think I know the answer.

JUST THE NIGHT BEFORE, I'D left Ralph in the care of my friend Evan while Aaron slept in our bedroom. I wanted to get a workout in, to sweat and move and take my mind off the fact that every day, my husband was slipping further and further away. I needed those deadlifts and snatches and kettlebell swings physically as much as I did mentally. The left side of Aaron's body was getting weaker and weaker. His left arm hung useless in a sling I bought for a couple dollars at the local pharmacy. His left leg was beginning to follow suit, dragging behind him and giving him the look of a very well-dressed zombie. He slept about twenty hours a day, and when I got home from work I'd grab his good hand like we were about to arm wrestle, hook my other arm under his armpit, and lift him up so he could hang out with us in the living room or the kitchen.

"Fucking pathetic," he'd say.

"No, you're not," I'd whisper, trying not to cry while we shuffled our way out of the bedroom.

"Not me!" he'd say. "You! You're still such a weakling! I weigh, like, thirty pounds and you can barely lift me!"

While I was up in the gym just working on my fitness, Aaron was having a violent seizure, crumbling to the floor in our living room while Evan served Ralph a second helping of macaroni and cheese. When Aaron woke, he insisted that Evan not call me at all. It would ruin my night, he insisted, I'd rush home instead of finishing my workout. Like any good friend, Evan didn't call me, but when I texted him to see how things were going, he spilled the beans and I drove home feeling stupid and selfish for prioritizing my mom butt over my dying husband. I found Aaron in the bathroom, where he'd asked Evan to leave him.

"Hey, Nornia," he said, smiling up at me from his slumped position against the bathtub, "how was your workout?"

He insisted he was fine, even after I cleaned him up and changed his clothes and put him to bed, his entire left side, from his face to his toes, almost completely paralyzed.

Aaron was not fine, but we told each other he was, just as we always had. I went downstairs to put in the laundry and called his doctor on the emergency line.

We affectionately referred to Aaron's oncologist as Dr. Mustache from day one. He has, as you may guess, facial hair that is downright Seussical, but that is the only whimsical thing about him. This man is a nerd, a brain tumor nerd, a man I like to imagine has one interest and one interest only: killing brain tumors. And, perhaps on weekends, building model train sets. If he's going to have an imaginary hobby, I want it to be something precise. Falconry would be a suitable alternative. Dr. Mustache has a collection of button-down shirts, each monogrammed with his initials. He speaks clearly and directly at every appointment, but to Aaron only, occasionally handing me a box of tissues in anticipation of bad news. It's nearly ten o'clock when I call him, and I imagine him in a clean, spare house somewhere on the south side of the city, perhaps eating a small bowl of cereal as a late-night snack. There is something about his voice—particularly its steady sternness— that gives me comfort, and makes me long for my father. I apologize for crying, and he tells me to wake up early tomorrow "or, whenever you want, really," and take Aaron to the ER. "I don't like this," he tells me, "we need to see what's going on."

"It isn't good," I tell him.

"No," he says, "it isn't."

I WAS RIGHT, AND SO was Dr. Mustache. An hour passes between when Aaron's MRI is over and when we actually see a doctor again. "Has anyone stopped in here yet? Like, a doctor?" the nurses ask repeatedly, and I remember this same dance from Halloween 2011, hours of waiting for the right person to deliver the news you don't want to hear. I hadn't been there when they'd told Aaron about his brain tumor. I had run home—to the bachelor pad of Aaron's that I'd just moved into—to grab the things you need for an unexpected night in the hospital: toothbrushes, pajamas, hoodies, basketball shorts, phone chargers, and warm socks. Our house had been filled with the evidence of the chaotic combination of our two lives. My mattress was still wedged into the kitchen, boxes of my books were stacked around the couch where a friend had crashed for the weekend, a pile of dirty dishes were half submerged in the cloudy water of our kitchen sink.

Where are you? Aaron had texted me as our friend drove my car from the highway and toward Aaron's hospital bed. *There's something I need to tell you.*

That's the thing about bad news: it wants to be told in person. Or, it usually does. My mother once sent me an email that read:

Subject: Your uncle
Is dead. Funeral soon. Call me?

The weight of Aaron's text sat with me on the long walk from the parking garage to his room, and when I walked into his room an audience of friends and family looked at me with eyes filled with tears and pity.

"I have a brain tumor," he said, gently tapping above his right eye, and I climbed right into his lap, disturbing cords and blankets until my forehead was pressed against his.

"They think it's small."

"Your brain?"

"The tumor."

"You'll be okay."

"I will, we will."

DR. MUSTACHE IS NOT IN, but his nurse practitioner, a grand-motherly figure with the appearance of a craft store enthusiast and the brain of a neuro-oncology genius, is unusually quiet when she parts the curtain to our room and steps in, his social worker just a few steps behind her. They both clean their hands with the antibacterial foam at the doorway. Sure, it's a required habit for medical professionals, but it still strikes me as funny— like they have some germ that will kill Aaron faster than the can-cer they're about to tell him is finally killing him. But it's habit, I'm sure, and also because you need to have something to do with your hands while you tell a person he is dying.

There is an art to the practice of telling a person that hospice is his only option. You may learn it from many years of motherhood as easily as you could through many years of an occupation deal-ing with death, but they've delivered this crushing news in a way that leaves Aaron and me feeling like this is a choice we've made, and not a death sentence we've been served.

"How do you feel?" his social worker, Margaret, asks him, and there is something about her, something so pure and good inside of her and her sweet voice, that we both begin to cry immediately, which is something we don't typically do. But then again, neither is being told Aaron is going to die.

"I'm not afraid to die," he tells her, "I just don't want to do it."

ONCE AARON HAS FINISHED HIS pancakes and I have finished my third cup of coffee, we go on with our lives. We pick up Ralph from day care, we feed him dinner, we watch a few hours of *Buffy the Vampire Slayer* and fall asleep holding hands.

I know for a fact that nobody cares about dreams but guess what? I'm going to tell you about a damn dream, okay? I dreamed my mother and I were caught in a flash flood that swept us up the street where I live, carrying us past parked cars and front yards that seemed untouched by the swell of water ripping down the street.

Just before we were washed clear across the park, my mother reached out and grabbed a rowboat and canoe from the curb of a neighbor's house. In defense of my neighborhood, this isn't actually how my neighbors store their watercraft, it's just one of those weird dream things. My mother took the rowboat, and I climbed into the canoe, where she tossed me a paddle and began to row her boat against the churning water, making slow progress toward my house.

I tried to follow, but paddling a canoe is a job for two, and I couldn't get myself turned in the right direction.

"I can't do it alone!" I cried, but she shook her head.

"Just paddle!" she shouted, and I felt my little vessel push back against the current trying to wash me away.

Acknowledgments

Thanks to my big dumb family for giving me a childhood that was both charmed and traumatizing. I almost forgive you for forgetting that I played the saxophone. But not quite.

My mother is the definition of a bad bitch. Madge, thank you for showing me how to be a woman, for always (eventually) forgiving me, and for loving me mostly unconditionally.

Aaron was the best thing ever to happen to me (sorry, Ralph) and I will carry him with me forever.

Steve taught me to love reading and writing; he was a ruthless editor even to a child. I think he would be proud of this book and also appalled at some of the content, which is about par for the relationship we had.

My best friend, Dave Gilmore, has been a thoughtful reader since 2001, and has picked me up off the ground more times than I can count. I'm sorry for when you tried to teach me guitar and for every time I picked the movie.

To the coven of women who are there for me every day, thank you.

It takes a whole damn village to raise a child, and I'm lucky to have one. If you watched Ralph so I could write, or go to yoga, or get drunk . . . thank you. If you read my blog or wrote me an email or hugged me in public; if you're my Internet troll: thank you. Haters are my motivators.

Julia Cheiffetz believed in me, and I'll always be grateful to have had her guidance and patience. Thank you for getting me, and for laughing at my jokes.

Jessica Regel is an actual angel. Look it up.

Dana, none of this would have happened if it weren't for you. Thank you.

Ralph, thank you for being on my team, and making me a mom. Please stop telling me not to sing or dance, it's starting to hurt my feelings.

About the author

Nora McInerny Purmort is the creator of a blog called My Husband's Tumor (listed on Tumblr's 'Big in 2014' list) and co-creator of her son Ralph, who she is currently raising to avenge his father's untimely death. Nora has been published in *The Washington Post*, *Glamour*, *USA Today* and *The Huffington Post*. She has also appeared on *The Today Show* and *All Things Considered*.

Twitter: @noraborealis.
Instagram: @noraborealis.
Visit myhusbandstumor.com.